The National Cancer Institute Clinical Trials Education Series

Cancer Clinical Trials Books

Cancer Clinical Trials: The Basic Workbook

The self-modulated workbook, with its accompanying activities, will help readers understand why cancer clinical trials are important, how they work, how participants' safety is protected, as well as some of the reasons so few adults participate in these trials. It is designed for individuals who want to develop a basic understanding of clinical trials.

Cancer Clinical Trials: The In-Depth Program

The textbook expands on the subjects outlined in *The Basic Workbook*. It features additional information on clinical trial design, resources for physician participation, and referral of individuals to studies. It is designed for health care professionals and others who seek a more in-depth understanding of clinical trials.

Cancer Clinical Trials: A Resource Guide For Outreach, Education, and Advocacy

The interactive workbook provides direction and guidance for individuals and organizations interested in developing specific clinical trial outreach and education activities. This guide can also be used along with either or both of the texts listed above.

Trainer's Guide for Cancer Education

A manual for planning and conducting educational sessions on cancer-related topics, including clinical trials.

Cancer Clinical Trials Resources

The following resources will help support cancer clinical trials education and outreach efforts.

Publications

Low literacy **brochures** on cancer clinical trials for potential participants:

- *If You Have Cancer...What You Should Know About Clinical Trials*

- *If You Have Cancer and Have Medicare...What You Should Know About Clinical Trials*

Clinical trial participant **booklets**:
- *Taking Part in Clinical Trials: What Cancer Patients Need to Know**
- *Taking Part in Clinical Trials: Cancer Prevention Studies—What Participants Need to Know**

*Also available in Spanish

Videos

- A clinical trial awareness video and speaker's guide, "Cancer Trials...Because Lives Depend on It"
- A video and discussion guide on deciding to take part in a clinical trial, "Cancer Clinical Trials: An Introduction for Patients and their Families"

Slide Programs

Three slide programs are available in PowerPoint on CD-ROM and on the *www.cancer.gov* Web site:

Cancer Clinical Trials: The Basics
Provides background on why cancer clinical trials are important, how they work, and how participants' safety is protected.

Cancer Clinical Trials: The Way We Make Progress Against Cancer
A brief community awareness presentation.

Cancer Clinical Trials: In-Depth Information
Expands on the subjects outlined above, featuring additional information on clinical trial design with resources for physician participation and referral of individuals to studies.

Ordering Information

To order these publications, contact the Cancer Information Service at 1-800-4-CANCER or log onto *www.cancer.gov/publications*. Most materials are available as PDF files on the Web site.

The Cancer Information Service
NCI's Cancer Information Service (CIS), with regional offices throughout the United States, may work with organizations and professionals to plan, implement, and evaluate culturally appropriate clinical trials education programs using the Clinical Trials Education Series. Contact the CIS at 1-800-4-CANCER.

Table of Contents

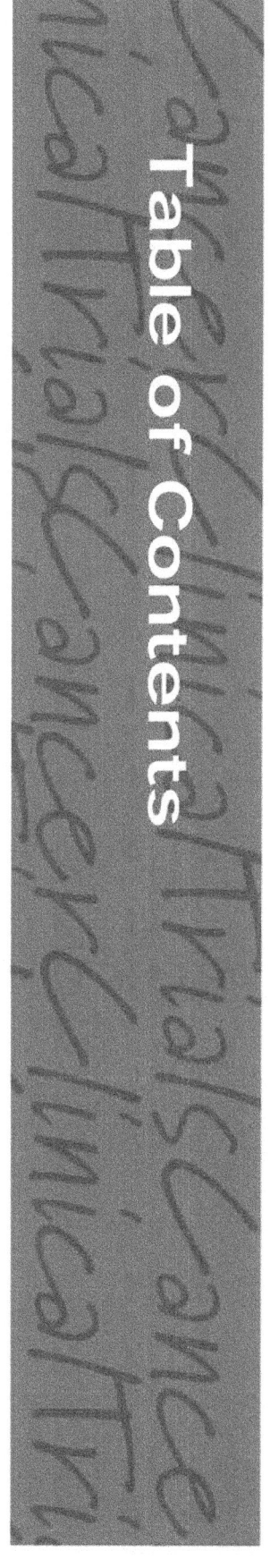

Preface

Research supports that the public understands very little about clinical trials. Some people are fearful of being "guinea pigs," even though participants in clinical trials receive high-quality care. Other people are not aware of clinical trials as an option, do not understand how they work, or do not have access to them.

Likewise, health care professionals may be unaware of appropriate clinical trials, may not want to refer people out of their practice, may believe that standard therapy is best, or may think that getting involved in clinical trials will add an undue administrative burden to their work.

Today's standard cancer treatments were yesterday's clinical trials. Successful clinical trials have:
- Increased survival rates of participants with testicular cancer, breast cancer, leukemia, and lymphoma
- Decreased morbidity associated with the surgical treatment of many cancers
- Resulted in the development of new compounds and techniques to reduce the side effects of cancer therapies

This guide is designed to familiarize health care professionals and others with the ins and outs of clinical trials. It describes how:
- The clinical trial process works
- Trials are designed to obtain particular information
- Clinical trials advance standard cancer treatment
- Trial participants are safeguarded
- People might face obstacles to participating in clinical trials
- To find a local clinical trial

After reading the guide and reviewing the case study, the reader will be better able to manage issues related to clinical trials. The reader should be able to:
- Discuss clinical trials as potential treatment or preventive options
- Answer people's questions and allay their fears about clinical trials
- Locate and refer people to accessible clinical trials
- Ultimately help advance the early detection, treatment, and eventual prevention of cancer

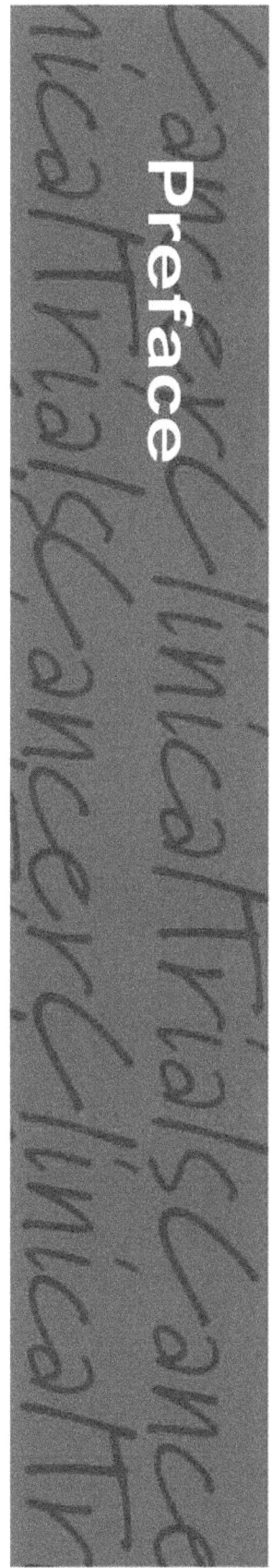

Introduction: An Overview of Clinical Trials

Approximately 555,550 people in the United States are expected to die of cancer each year—an average of more than 1,500 people a day. As the second leading cause of death after heart disease, cancer accounts for one in four deaths each year. Moreover, about 1,284,900 new cancer cases are expected to be diagnosed in 2002. As widespread as the threat of cancer is among all Americans, its impact is felt disproportionately by racial and ethnic minorities, the medically underserved, and people over age 65.

Scientific research continues to provide valuable insights into the causes of cancer. But research is an incremental process, moving forward in small, carefully planned steps. Advances typically begin with basic research in the laboratory. After years of testing in cells and tissues, promising leads are tested in animal models of human cancers. Only after treatments or techniques prove successful in animals can they be evaluated in people through clinical trials. Well-designed, well-run clinical trials are the only way to determine the true effectiveness of a promising new agent or intervention being investigated.

Clinical trials are designed to answer specific questions about the effects of a therapy or technique designed to improve human health. The trials are planned in advance, follow a rigorous scientific process, and the findings are analyzed. The scientific process has built-in safeguards for participants, who are selected carefully from volunteers. Clinical trials are usually conducted in a progressive series of steps, called phases. The process starts with small trials testing the safety of an intervention and moves to progressively larger trials. The larger trials compare the effectiveness of the new intervention given to the investigational group to the currently accepted standard care given to the control group.

Clinical trials are mechanisms for developing better methods of detecting, treating, and eventually preventing diseases like cancer. The enormous strides made in treating childhood cancer, for

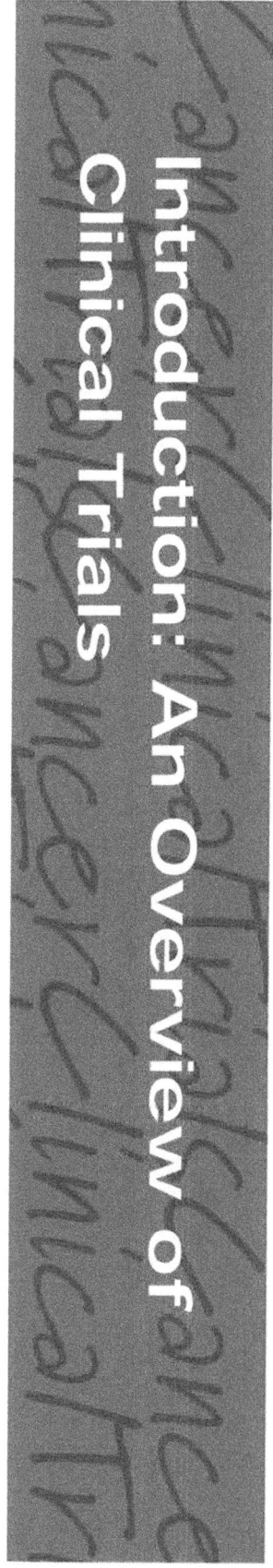

example, are the direct result of clinical trials. In the United States today, more than 70 percent of children with cancer live at least 5 years after diagnosis, as opposed to only 55 percent in the mid-1970s.

More than 60 percent of children with cancer participate in clinical trials, yet only 3 percent of adults with cancer do. To answer the most pressing questions about cancer—and to do so quickly—many more adults must participate in clinical trials. To encourage participation, the National Cancer Institute (NCI) and other organizations provide information to ensure that health care professionals and the people they treat understand clinical trials, consider them as an option, and can easily locate them in their communities. Clinical trials should not be considered only in terms of caring for people who have cancer. They may also present prevention and early detection options for people at high risk of developing cancer.

For more basic information about clinical trials, see "Facts and Figures about Cancer Clinical Trials" at *http://www.cancer.gov/clinicaltrials/facts-and-figures.*

1
The Clinical Trial Process

Learning Objectives
- Identify the steps in the drug development process
- Name the various types and phases of clinical trials
- Describe special access programs

The Drug Development and Approval Process

Clinical trials are a key part of the drug development and approval process. The entire process takes place under the watchful eye of the Food and Drug Administration (FDA). As a consumer protection agency of the U.S. Department of Health and Human Services, FDA is required by law to review all test results for new drugs to ensure that they are safe and effective for specific uses. "Safe" does not mean that the product is free of possible adverse side effects; rather, it means that its potential benefits outweigh any known risks. The FDA approval process is focused on drugs, but similar processes exist for the approval of:
- New devices (e.g., infusion pumps)
- Agents (e.g., vitamins and medications)
- Biologics (e.g., vaccines)

For purposes of illustration, the process outlined in this text focuses on drug approval.

Before a new drug or biologic agent that shows promising results in the lab can be tested in people, its sponsor must submit an Investigational New Drug (IND) application to FDA. Once the application is approved, the sponsor can begin testing the drug in clinical trials with human participants. If these trials demonstrate that the new drug is safe and superior to standard treatment, the sponsor can file a New Drug Application (NDA) or a Biologics

Steps in the Drug Development Process

1. **Early research and preclinical testing.** During early research and preclinical testing, drugs undergo basic laboratory investigation and animal model testing for efficacy and toxicity. This step takes about 4 years.

2. **Investigational New Drug application.** The trial sponsor files an IND application with FDA. If FDA approves the application, clinical trials begin.

3. **Phase 1 clinical trial.** Phase 1 trials determine the safety and appropriate dosage of the drug for humans. It might take about 2 years before enough participants enroll in the trial. If phase 1 trials are successful, researchers design phase 2 trials.

4. **Phase 2 clinical trial.** Phase 2 trials evaluate the effectiveness of the drug and look for side effects. It might take up to 2 years to enroll participants for these trials. If phase 2 trials are successful, researchers design phase 3 trials.

5. **Phase 3 clinical trial.** Phase 3 trials evaluate the effectiveness of the new treatment, compared with standard treatment. It might take 3 to 4 years to enroll enough participants for these trials. Researchers report trial results in peer-reviewed scientific journals and at professional meetings.

6. **New Drug Application.** The trial sponsor files an NDA or BLA with FDA. The sponsor submits this application to FDA once it has adequate data to support a certain indication for a drug (usually by finding that the drug is safe and superior to standard treatment in a definitive phase 3 trial).

7. **FDA approval.** FDA approves the claim that is being made about the drug, which takes about 1½ years. After approval, it can be marketed to the public. FDA approval allows the drug to be "labeled" for a specific use. This label includes information on the drug's dosage, indications, safety, and side effects.

License Application (BLA) to FDA. Only after FDA approves the drug can it be marketed.

For an overview of the drug approval process from start to finish, see FDA's *From Test Tube to Patient: New Drug Development in the United States*. This book tells the story of new drug development in the United States and highlights the consumer protection role of FDA. Call 1-888-INFO-FDA or see the Web site *http://www.fda.gov*.

Types and Phases of Clinical Trials

Cancer clinical trials focus on developing new strategies for the prevention, detection, treatment, and overall improvement of the care and quality of life of people with cancer or people at high risk for developing cancer. In cancer research, a clinical trial is designed to show how a particular anticancer strategy affects the people who receive it.

Clinical trials differ by type and phase, but they all involve rigorous scientific testing. Each type of clinical trial attempts to answer different research questions:

- **Prevention trials:** What kinds of interventions—such as lifestyle modifications, dietary supplements, or drugs—can prevent cancer from occurring?
- **Screening and early detection trials:** What tests can find cancer as early as possible in healthy people?
- **Diagnostic trials:** How can new tests or procedures identify a suspected cancer earlier or more accurately?
- **Genetics trials:** Can gene-transfer therapy be used to treat cancer?
- **Treatment trials:** What new interventions (e.g., drugs, biologics, surgical procedures, radiation) can help people who have cancer?
- **Quality-of-life and supportive care trials:** What kinds of interventions can improve the comfort and quality of life of people who have cancer?

Clinical trials occur in four phases, each of which is designed to answer different research questions:

- **Phase 1:** How does the treatment affect the human body? How should the treatment be given? What dosage is safe?
- **Phase 2:** Does the treatment do what it is supposed to do for a particular cancer? How does the treatment affect the human body?
- **Phase 3:** Is the new treatment (or new use of a treatment) better than current practice?
- **Phase 4:** What are the effects of an approved treatment?

The phases of clinical trials are explained in the context of drug treatment trials on the pages that follow. But the same concepts apply to most types of clinical trials, which are described after treatment trials.

	Phase 1	Phase 2	Phase 3	Phase 4
Number of participants	15–30 people	Fewer than 100 people	Generally, from 100 to thousands of people	Several hundred to several thousand people
Purpose	• To find a safe dosage • To decide how the agent should be given • To observe how the agent affects the human body	• To determine if the agent or intervention has an effect on a particular cancer • To see how the agent or intervention affects the human body	• To compare the new agent or intervention (or new use of a treatment) with the current standard	• To further evaluate the long-term safety and effectiveness of a new treatment

Treatment Trials

Treatment trials are designed to test the safety and effectiveness of new drugs, biological agents, techniques, or other interventions in people who have been diagnosed with cancer. These trials evaluate the potential clinical usefulness of a therapy or compare an investigational treatment against standard treatment, if there is one.

Phase 1

Phase 1 trials are the first step in transforming laboratory data into clinical care. While the primary goal of a phase 1 trial is to determine the toxic effects, pharmacological behavior, and recommended dosage of a therapy or technique for future trials, these trials are conducted with therapeutic intent.

In a phase 1 trial, the study participants (usually less than 30 people) are divided into cohorts of three to six participants. Each cohort of participants is treated with an increased dose of the new therapy or technique. Results in early participants greatly influence the dose subsequent participants receive. Initial dosage is based on preclinical testing and is usually quite conservative. If no serious side effects are seen in the initial group after a period of time, usually 3 to 4 weeks, the next group of participants receives a higher dose. This pattern is repeated until a certain percentage of participants experience dose-limiting toxicity—that is, side effects strong enough that the next group of participants should not get a higher dose. The highest dose with acceptable toxicity is determined to be appropriate for further testing.

Phase 1 trials are not limited to "first in human" studies. Subsequent phase 1 trials often evaluate new schedules or combinations of established drugs or radiation. Later phase 1 trials may also be conducted to evaluate toxicity, response, and pharmacokinetics in populations that might not have been included in prior trials, such as children or the elderly. Some phase 1 trials are pilot trials for larger trials designed to determine the interaction of a drug with another treatment or substance.

Who Participates

Almost all phase 1 trials of new anticancer drugs involve participants with a cancer that lacks or does not respond to standard treatment. People with many types of cancer can participate in the same phase 1 trial. Participants are generally required to have organ function capable of metabolizing and excreting the drug and a 1- to 2-month life expectancy, in order to evaluate the drug's effects and the body's response to it.

Possible Benefits

- If the new agent under study has an effect on the cancer, participants may be among the first to benefit.

Possible Risks

- Because phase 1 trials are often the first studies involving humans, unpredictable side effects can occur.

Phase 2

Phase 2 trials are designed to evaluate the effectiveness of the drug in a somewhat larger group of participants (usually less than 100), using the dosage determined to be safe in phase 1 trials. On the basis of their findings in phase 1 trials, researchers often focus phase 2 trials on cancers for which no effective treatment exists and/or that are most likely to show a response to therapy. In choosing which type of cancer to study, researchers may also take into account effective alternatives and choose a cancer that has none. Some anticancer compounds being developed target molecular pathways in specific cancers, a development that may affect the cancers chosen for phase 2 trials.

In most phase 2 trials, all participants receive the same dose of the drug (or undergo the same intervention). The new treatment is assessed for effectiveness, and additional safety information is noted. Even if the new treatment seems effective, it usually requires further testing before entering widespread use. Because the treatment has not been compared with any other therapy or technique, its relative value is unclear, and it is impossible to rule out other factors that may have influenced its effectiveness. In addition, phase 2 trials are often too short to determine long-term benefits; larger and longer phase 3 trials are more suited to this purpose.

Some phase 2 trials compare different schedules of administering the same drug. At the end of such trials, the most promising regimen is chosen to move into phase 3 trials. Participants in this type of phase 2 trial are assigned at random to either the investigational group, which is given the new treatment, or the control group, which receives the standard treatment. Neither the participants nor their doctors choose which group individual participants will be in.

Who Participates

Generally, people who take part in phase 2 trials have not found the current standard of care effective or have cancers for which there is no standard treatment. Participants are generally required to have adequate organ function, a 3-month life expectancy, and a limited number of prior treatments.

Possible Benefits

- If the new agent has an effect on the cancer, participants may be among the first to benefit.

Possible Risks

- Unpredictable side effects may occur.

Phase 3

Phase 3 trials are large trials (usually involving more than 100 participants) designed to determine whether a new therapy or technique is more effective or less debilitating than a standard treatment. These trials are conducted at multiple institutions around the country, including community settings. Because the results of phase 3 trials guide health care professionals and people with cancer in making treatment decisions, their results should apply to aspects such as survival time and quality of life.

Like phase 2 trials, phase 3 trials usually focus on specific types of cancer. Participants enrolling in a phase 3 trial are assigned at random to an investigational group, which is given the new treatment, or a control group, which receives the current standard treatment. Some trials can also include more than two study groups, depending on the research questions being asked.

Who Participates

Many people with cancer get their first treatment in a phase 3 trial. Eligibility requirements vary with the disease stage or other factors being studied. Phase 3 trials typically involve large numbers of participants in order to determine true effectiveness.

Possible Benefits

- Regardless of the group a participant is assigned to, he or she will receive at a minimum the best widely accepted standard treatment.
- If a participant is taking the new treatment and it is shown to work, he or she may be among the first to benefit.

Possible Risks

- New treatments under study are not always better than, or even as good as, standard treatment.
- New treatments may have side effects that are worse than those of standard treatment.
- Despite phase 1 and 2 testing, unexpected side effects may occur.
- If the new treatment has benefits, it still may not work for every participant (just as standard treatments do not help everyone).
- Participants receiving the standard treatment may not benefit as much as those receiving the new one.

Finding Out About Standard Cancer Care

Standard cancer care is the accepted and widely used treatment for a certain type of cancer. It is based on the results of past research. The National Cancer Institute's Web site *www.cancer.gov* contains a database of the latest information about cancer and clinical trials. Specialists review current literature from more than 70 medical journals, evaluate its relevance, and synthesize it into clear summaries for the public and health professionals. Many of the summaries are also available in Spanish.

Phase 4

Phase 4 trials are used to further evaluate the long-term safety and effectiveness of a treatment. Less common than phase 1, 2, and 3 trials, phase 4 trials usually take place after the new treatment has been approved for standard use.

Other Types of Trials
Adjuvant and Neoadjuvant Treatment Trials

Adjuvant trials are additional therapy after standard treatment. They are designed to prevent the recurrence of cancer in people who no longer show clinical evidence of disease. Adjuvant trials attempt to treat the subclinical or microscopic disease thought to be responsible for cancer recurrence and therefore improve disease-free and overall survival. The combination of standard and adjuvant treatments is initially tested in a small feasibility or pilot study similar to a single-agent phase 2 trial. This is followed by a randomized phase 3 trial if the combination proves safe and effective.

Neoadjuvant trials are additional therapy before standard treatment. These trials evaluate treatments designed to reduce tumor size to a point where it can be definitively treated by therapies that are considered the best standard treatment. For example, clinical trials have shown that chemotherapy can reduce an inoperable breast cancer to a size that can be removed surgically.

Both adjuvant and neoadjuvant trials are phased like other treatment protocols, with the phase dependent on the major objective of the trial.

Who Participates

People who have no clinical evidence of disease after primary treatment, but who are at high risk of recurrence, participate in adjuvant trials. People whose cancer, once reduced, could be effectively treated by therapies considered the best standard treatment participate in neoadjuvant trials.

Prevention Trials

Cancer prevention trials are designed for people at risk of developing cancer. The trials evaluate the safety and effectiveness of various risk-reduction strategies. The two types of prevention trials answer the following questions:

- **Action trials:** Can a person's actions—such as exercising more or quitting smoking—prevent cancer?
- **Agent trials:** Can taking certain medicines, vitamins, minerals, or food supplements lower the risk of certain types of cancer? (Agent trials are also known as chemoprevention trials.)

Chemoprevention trials compare a promising new prevention agent or technique with a standard agent or technique, or placebo. The investigational group takes the agent being studied; the control group takes either the standard agent that is being compared with the study agent or—because there may be no standard agent—a look-alike agent that contains no active ingredient, called a placebo.

Who Participates

Prevention trials seek participants from various age groups and socioeconomic backgrounds or people who have combinations of cancer risk factors. Participants in prevention trials are otherwise healthy individuals who are at risk for cancer.

Possible Benefits

- If the intervention being studied is found to be effective, participants may be among the first to benefit.

Possible Risks

- New cancer prevention interventions may have unknown side effects or risks.
- The drug intervention may have worse side effects or be less effective than standard preventive measures.
- Even if a new drug or intervention is effective, it may not work for every participant.

Screening Trials

Screening trials assess the effectiveness of new means of detecting the earliest stages of cancer. In addition, these trials examine whether early treatment improves overall survival or disease-free survival. Screening tools include imaging tests and laboratory tests.

Who Participates

Participants are healthy and may be chosen to represent particular age groups or socioeconomic backgrounds. Screening trials also seek participants with certain cancer risk factors, such as belonging to a family that has a genetic predisposition to cancer.

Possible Benefits

- For many types of cancer, detecting the disease at an early stage can result in earlier treatment and an improved outcome.
- Screening trials often encourage participants to continue screening on a regular basis, which can lead to improved health overall.
- Screening trials for people with a genetic predisposition to cancer can alert other family members to begin regular cancer screening, aid in early detection, and help in the diagnosis and treatment of potential cancers.

Possible Risks

- Some of the imaging procedures used in screening may be uncomfortable or require participants to be in confined spaces for some period of time.
- If an imaging technique is being studied, participants may be exposed to x-rays or radioactive substances.
- Tests can be time consuming.

Diagnostic Trials

Diagnostic trials develop better tools for physicians to use in classifying types and phases of cancer, and in managing the care of people with cancer. Some trials compare the ability of two diagnostic techniques to provide information about a suspected cancer. Genetic tests are being evaluated as diagnostic tools to classify cancers further, thus helping physicians direct cancer therapy and improve treatments for people with specific genetic mutations. Diagnostic trials may also evaluate techniques designed to measure and monitor cancer response more accurately or less invasively, such as using a new imaging tool that eliminates the need for surgery.

Who Participates

Participants include people with cancer or symptoms suggesting cancer.

Possible Benefits

- The diagnostic test under investigation may be better and less invasive than current tests.
- A new diagnostic tool may help detect cancer recurrence, which could lead to improved outcomes.

Possible Risks

- Participation in a diagnostic trial may require people to take multiple tests.

Genetics Trials

Actual genetic intervention (such as gene-transfer) trials are few in number, however trials are under way where actual cellular manipulation at the gene level occurs. Most genetics research involves looking at tissue or blood samples from large populations of people in order to determine how genetic make-up can influence detection, diagnosis, prognosis, and treatment. This genetic epidemiologic research does not involve any actual intervention. Rather, it is designed to broaden understanding of the causes of cancer. Genetics research is also being used to develop targeted treatments based on the genetics of a tumor. Genetics research is a critical component of cancer research because it helps scientists understand the causes of cancer and can lead to developing clinical trials for the prevention, detection, and treatment of cancer.

Quality-of-Life and Supportive Care Trials

Quality-of-life and supportive care trials test interventions designed to improve quality of life for people with cancer and their families. They seek better therapies or psychosocial interventions for people experiencing nutrition problems, infection, pain, nausea and vomiting, sleep disorders, depression, and other effects of cancer or its treatment. Some supportive care trials target families and caregivers to help them cope. The effectiveness of supportive care trials may be measured either:

- **Subjectively:** Is the person's pain reduced?
- **Objectively:** Are the white blood cell counts improved?

Who Participates

Participants include:

- People who are interested in relief from the effects of cancer or its treatment
- Family members or others who want support in caregiving or meeting their own needs

Possible Benefits

- If the intervention is found to be effective, a person with cancer and his or her family may be among the first to benefit.

Possible Risks

- People may not benefit from participating in the trial.

Special Access Programs

Investigational drugs may be made available for use outside of a clinical trial. Working with NCI and other sponsors, FDA has established special conditions under which a person with cancer can receive unapproved cancer drugs that have shown clinical benefit.

Group C

In the 1970s, NCI researchers became concerned about the time it took to bring to market investigational drugs found to have antitumor activity. Working with FDA, NCI established the "Group C" classification to allow access to drugs with reproducible activity. Group C agents are investigational drugs provided by the National Cancer Institute to properly trained physicians for the treatment of individual patients who meet specific eligibility criteria within this category and are treated according to a protocol.

Each Group C drug protocol specifies eligibility, reporting methodology, and drug use. Group C designation speeds new drugs to people who need them most. The process allows NCI to gather important information on the safety as well as activity of the drugs in the settings where they will be most used after FDA approval. Drugs are placed in the Group C category by agreement between FDA and NCI. Group C drugs are always provided free of charge, and the Centers for Medicare and Medicaid Services (formerly the Health Care Financing Administration) provides coverage for its beneficiaries for care associated with Group C therapy.

Treatment IND

In 1987, FDA began authorizing the use of new drugs still in the development process to treat certain seriously ill people. In these cases, the process is referred to as a treatment Investigational New Drug (IND) application. Clinical trials of the new drug must already be under way and have demonstrated positive results.

FDA sets guidelines about:

- What serious and life-threatening illnesses constitute
- How much must be known about a drug's side effects and benefits
- Where physicians can obtain the drug for treatment

For many seriously ill people, the possible benefits outweigh the risks associated with taking an unapproved drug.

Less common ways that people can receive investigational drugs are through expanded access protocols or mechanisms known as special or compassionate exception.

Expanded Access Protocols

Expanded access protocols are available for a limited number of well-studied investigational drugs awaiting final FDA approval. Expanded access allows a wider group of people to be treated with a drug. The purpose is to make investigational drugs that have significant activity against specific cancers available before the FDA approval process has been completed.

The IND sponsor must apply to FDA to make the drug available through an expanded access protocol. There must be enough evidence from completed trials to show that the drug may be effective to treat a specific type of cancer and that it does not have unreasonable risks. FDA generally approves expanded access only if no other satisfactory treatments are available for the disease.

Special or Compassionate Exception

People who do not meet the eligibility criteria for a clinical trial of an investigational drug may be eligible to receive the drug. The person's doctor contacts the trial sponsor and provides the person's medical information and treatment history; requests are evaluated on a case-by-case basis. FDA must approve each request to provide the drug outside a clinical trial. There should be reasonable expectation that the drug will prolong survival or improve quality of life.

Considerations when determining whether a person may receive an investigational drug as a special exception include:

- Is the person ineligible for a clinical trial?
- Have standard therapies been exhausted?
- Is there objective evidence that the investigational agent is effective for the person's type of disease?
- Can the drug potentially benefit the person?
- What is the risk to the person?

In some cases, even people who qualify might not be able to obtain the drug if it is in limited quantity and high demand.

Refer to the case study in section 7, page 73, for a review and summary of content covered in this workbook.

2
Clinical Trial Design and Interpretation of Results

Learning Objectives
- Define key members of the research team
- Review key components of a clinical trial
- Describe the purpose of the randomization, stratification, and blinding in clinical trial protocols
- Name common statistical methods used to interpret clinical trial results

Clinical trials follow strict scientific guidelines that dictate how a study is designed and who participates in it. The reasons for these guidelines may not be immediately clear to a person urgently seeking treatment, but they protect people and provide scientifically sound results that can lead to truly effective therapies and techniques.

Research Team Members

Designing and implementing a clinical trial requires the many talents of a multidisciplinary research team. Each team may be set up differently, depending on an institution's policy and resources. Typical team members and their responsibilities include:

- **Principal investigator**—oversees all aspects of a clinical trial, specifically, concept development; protocol writing; protocol submission for institutional review board (IRB) approval; participant recruitment; informed consent; and data collection, analysis, interpretation, and presentation.

- **Research nurse**—coordinates the clinical trial and educates staff, participants, and referring health care providers. This nurse acts as an information conduit from the clinical setting to the principal investigator and vice versa, and assists the principal investigator with toxicity and response monitoring, quality assurance, audits, and data management and analysis.

- **Data manager**—handles the management of clinical trial data, including electronic data entry. Collaborates with the principal investigator and research nurse to identify what participant data will be tracked. The data manager also provides data to monitoring agencies and prepares summaries for interim and final data analysis.

- **Staff physicians and nurses**—administer treatment to participants as specified in the protocol; assess and record toxicity, drug tolerance, and adverse events; collaborate with the principal investigator and research nurse in observing and reporting clinical trends; and provide clinical management and participant education.

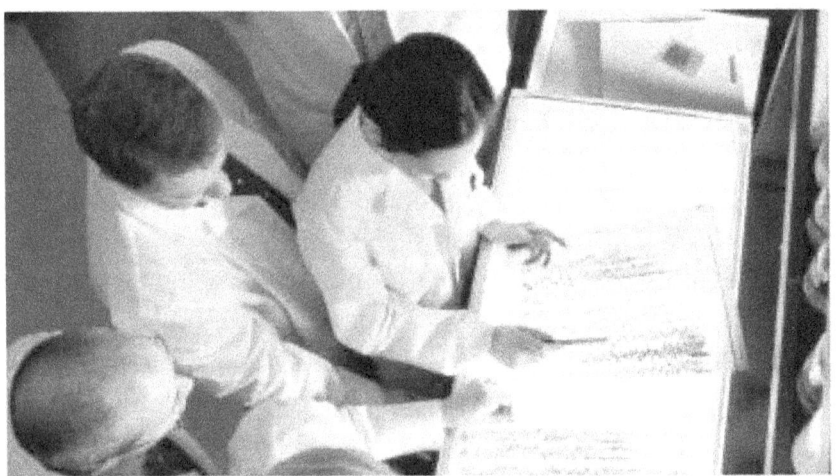

Components of a Clinical Trial

Protocol

Every trial has a written, detailed action plan called a protocol. The protocol provides the background, specifies the objectives, and describes the design and organization of the trial. Every site participating in the trial uses the same protocol, ensuring consistency of procedures and enhancing communication. This uniformity ensures that results from all sites can be combined and compared.

The clinical trial protocol answers the following questions:
* What is the scientific rationale or basis for conducting the trial?
* What are the objectives?
* How many participants will be in the trial?
* Who is eligible to participate? (This is determined on the basis of factors such as age and disease status.)
* What is the intervention, and what is its duration or schedule?
* What side effects might there be?
* What medical tests or followup visits will participants have? How often?
* What information will be gathered about participants?
* What are the endpoints of the trial?

The following FDA-required protocol elements help investigators answer the questions above and assist participants and health care professionals in understanding the goals of a clinical trial:

- General information
- Background information (with relevant references from the scientific literature)
- Trial objectives and purpose
- Trial design
- Participant selection and withdrawal
- Participant treatment
- Efficacy assessment
- Safety assessment
- Statistics
- Direct access to source data and documents
- Quality control and quality assurance
- Ethics
- Data handling and record keeping
- Financing and insurance
- Publication policy
- Supplements

Eligibility Criteria

Participant eligibility criteria can range from general (age, sex, type of cancer) to specific (prior treatment, tumor characteristics, blood cell counts, organ function). Eligibility criteria may also vary with trial phase. In phase 1 and 2 trials, the criteria often focus on making sure that people who might be harmed because of abnormal organ function or other factors are not put at risk. Phase 2 and 3 trials often add criteria regarding disease type and stage, and number of prior treatments.

Eligibility criteria might be very detailed if researchers think that a drug will work best on a specific type of cancer or population. Trials with narrow eligibility criteria might be complicated to conduct and might produce less widely applicable results.

Researchers therefore attempt to include as many types of people as possible in a clinical trial without making the study population too diverse to tell whether the treatment might be as effective on a more narrowly defined population. The more diverse the trial's population, the more useful the results could be to the general population, particularly in phase 3 trials. Results of phase 3 trials should be as generally applicable as possible in order to benefit the maximum number of people.

The trend today is toward broadening eligibility criteria for phase 3 clinical trials. Less restrictive criteria may enable more researchers and people with cancer to participate in these trials. With more participants, the disadvantages of having a more diverse population will be outweighed by the results applying more generally to the population.

Endpoints

An endpoint is a measurable outcome that indicates an intervention's effectiveness. Endpoints differ depending on the phase and type of trial. For instance, a treatment trial endpoint could be tumor response or participant survival. Quality-of-life or supportive care trial endpoints could include participants' welfare and control of symptoms.

Examples of endpoints include:
- **Tumor response rate**—the proportion of trial participants whose tumor was reduced in size by a specific amount, usually described as a percentage. If 7 of 10 patients responded, the response rate is 70 percent.
- **Disease–free survival**—the amount of time a participant survives without cancer occurring or recurring, usually measured in months.
- **Overall survival**—the amount of time a participant lives, typically measured from the beginning of the clinical trial until the time of death.

Tumor response rate is a typical endpoint in a phase 2 treatment trial. However, even if a treatment reduces the size of a participant's tumor and lengthens the period of disease-free survival, it may not lengthen overall survival. In such a case, side effects and failure to extend overall survival might outweigh the benefit of longer disease-free survival. Alternatively, the participant's improved quality of life during the tumor-free interval might outweigh other factors.

Because tumor response rates are often temporary and may not translate into long-term survival benefits for the participant, response rate is a reasonable measure of a treatment's effectiveness in a phase 2 trial, whereas participant survival and quality of life are better endpoints in a phase 3 trial.

Randomization

In phase 3 trials (and some phase 2 trials) participants are assigned to either the investigational or control group by chance, via a computer program or table of random numbers. This process, called randomization, gives each person the same chance of being assigned to either group. Randomization ensures that unknown factors do not influence the trial results.

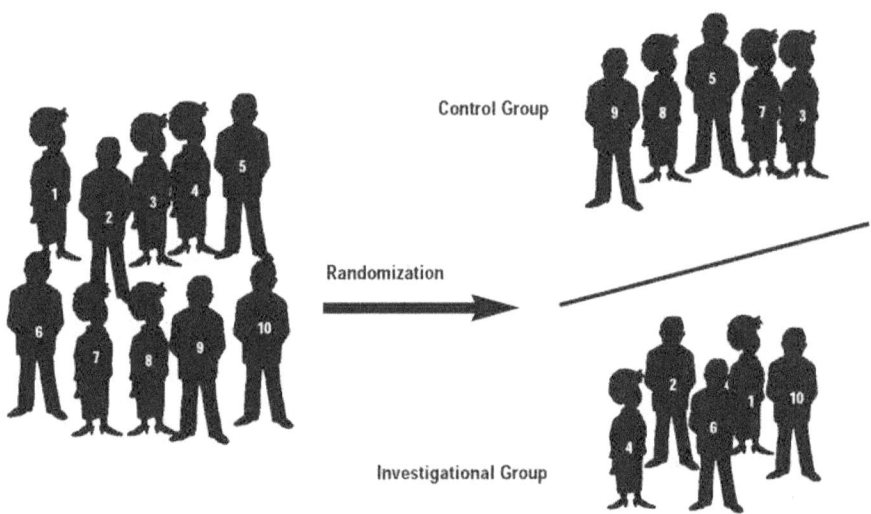

Randomization is a method used to prevent bias in research. A computer or a table of random numbers generates treatment assignments, and participants have an equal chance to be assigned to one of two or more groups (e.g., the control group or the investigational group).

If physicians or participants themselves chose the group, assignments might be biased. Physicians, for instance, might unconsciously assign participants with a more hopeful prognosis to the experimental group, thus making the new therapy seem more effective than it really is. Conversely, participants with a less hopeful prognosis might pick the experimental treatment, leading it to look less effective than it really is.

Randomization tends to produce comparable groups in terms of factors affecting prognosis and other participant characteristics. In this way, randomization guarantees the validity of the conclusion concerning the effectiveness of the treatment.

Stratification

Stratification is used in randomized trials when factors that can influence the intervention's success are known. For instance, participants whose cancer has spread from the original tumor site

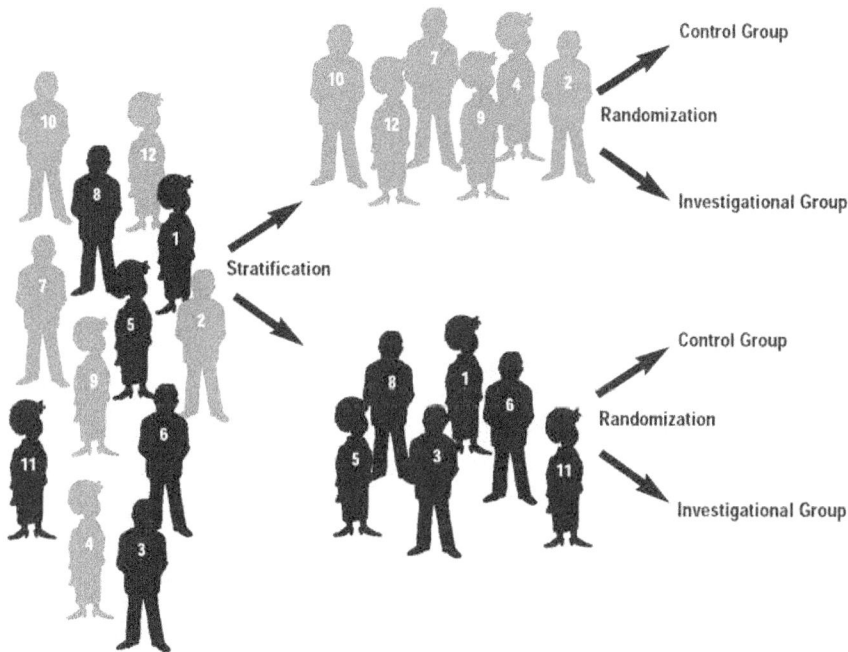

Stratification is a process used in randomized trials when factors that can influence the intervention's success are known. Assignment of interventions within the two groups is then randomized. Stratification enables researchers to look in separate subgroups to see whether differences exist.

can be separated, or stratified, from those whose cancer has not spread. Assignment of interventions within the two groups is then randomized. Stratification enables researchers to look at factors in both groups.

Blinding

Trials set so that participants do not know which intervention they are receiving are known as single-blinded trials. Those in which neither researchers nor participants know who is in the investigational or control group are called double-blinded trials. Double-blinded trials ensure that people assessing the outcome will not be influenced by knowing which intervention a participant is receiving and also that ancillary followup treatment will be the same.

Data Collection and Management Tools

Most research teams use standardized and newly created tools to collect, process, analyze, and audit data. Tools vary in format from visual analog scales to open-ended questionnaires. Examples of tools for participants to use to self-report data include diaries, calendars, logs, and surveys.

The case report form is the basic tool of data abstraction. Many reports use a Web-based format, others are paper-based. NCI is constructing an informatics system that will reduce the extensive paperwork often associated with clinical trials. For example, the Common Toxicity Criteria (CTC), a Web-based, interactive application, uses standardized language to identify and grade adverse events in cancer clinical trials. Forms are also available for rapid reporting of adverse events, electronically or by telephone, to alert researchers to potential safety issues. The Adverse Event Expedited Reporting System (AdEERS) is a Web-based program that enables researchers using NCI-sponsored investigational agents to expedite the reporting of serious and/or unexpected adverse events directly to NCI and FDA.

Using Statistics to Interpret Results

Researchers use statistical methods to determine whether an effect observed in a clinical trial is real (statistically significant) or caused by chance (not statistically significant). Although the examples included here use terminology and illustrations from treatment trials, these statistical techniques apply to all types of clinical trials.

Key Terms

Familiarity with the following terms is useful in understanding how researchers use statistics to interpret clinical trial results:

- **p-values** reflect the likelihood that the results of a clinical trial are because of chance rather than due to a real difference between the tested treatments. The smaller the value of p, the greater the likelihood that the results are not because of chance. A p-value of 0.05 (that is, 1 in 20) or smaller is widely accepted as an indication that the results are statistically significant.
- **Confidence intervals** reflect a range of values of the true value that would be obtained if everyone with a particular cancer were treated with the treatment under study. The wider the interval, the more variable the result and the less likely it is to be close to the true value. Confidence intervals are typically thought of as the approximate bounds or limits of the true value. Researchers frequently use either a 95 or a 99 percent confidence interval.
- **Sample size** is the number of people participating in a trial.
- **Statistical power** refers to the chance of finding a statistically significant result when there is one. Ideally, statistical power should be 0.80 or 0.90—reflecting an 80 to 90 percent chance of detecting that the true difference in treatment effectiveness is the smallest size considered medically important to detect.
- **Relative risk** is the likelihood that cancer will occur within a specific timeframe in one group versus another.

Statistical Significance

The result of a clinical trial can be statistically significant (not due to chance) without being clinically significant (medically important). Suppose, for instance, that a group receiving an experimental treatment has a 2 percent higher survival rate than the group receiving the standard treatment. This difference could be statistically significant, but if participants who survive longer experience serious side effects, it may not be medically important. In this case, the side effects might be worth tolerating only if the experimental treatment group has a 10 percent higher survival rate. Good trial planning and interpretation take into consideration both medical importance and statistical significance.

The results of a trial are usually considered statistically significant when data comparison results in a p-value of 0.05 or smaller. If the p-value is 0.01 or even 0.001, the results are considered even more significant because there is less likelihood that the results are due to chance.

Confidence intervals are often useful data for researchers because they enable researchers to generalize the results of the trial to the population.

For example, in a treatment trial with an investigational and a control group, the mean (average) values of the endpoints (e.g., survival for 5 years after treatment) are calculated separately for each group. Then the standard error—how far the values extend on either side of the mean—is calculated for each group. The less overlap between the confidence interval for the standard treatment group and the experimental treatment group, the more likely the difference between the groups is statistically significant. Research reports typically include confidence intervals, for example:

> The rate of 5-year survival for group A was 73 percent (95% confidence interval, 65.7% to 80.3%). The rate of 5-year survival for group B was 58 percent (95% confidence interval, 49.8% to 66.2%). $p = 0.004$.

In this case, the confidence intervals come close to each other—65.7 percent and 66.2 percent—but do not overlap. The *p*-value is definitely statistically significant.

Confidence intervals can give an indication of whether the results of small-sized trials that are not statistically significant are nevertheless medically significant. They can be particularly important tools when the trial size is limited because the type of cancer is rare.

Trial Size

The number of participants in a clinical trial greatly influences its statistical significance. With too few participants, a trial does not generate enough information to draw a conclusion, and important results may be missed. On the other hand, by testing more people than needed to obtain statistically significant results, a trial takes longer to produce results and may give ineffective or unsafe therapy to more people than necessary.

When planning a clinical trial, researchers first decide how large a difference between treatment groups is medically important. Next, they calculate sample size, or how many people should be enrolled in the trial. The sample should include enough participants to get a statistically significant result (a *p*-value of 0.05 or smaller).

Sample size also influences the statistical power of the research and is calculated before the trial begins. As sample size increases, statistical power increases. Ideally, power should be 0.80 or 0.90. Calculating statistical power helps a researcher decide how many people to enroll in a trial.

Relative Risk

Relative risk usually describes the risk of getting cancer based on lifestyle, environmental exposure to cancer-causing agents, or family history of disease. However, when used in cancer clinical trial reports, relative risk usually indicates the likelihood that cancer will occur within a specific timeframe in one group versus another.

Intention to Treat

Phase 3 trials are often analyzed on an intention-to-treat basis—that is, all participants who were initially admitted into the trial and randomized are included in the primary analysis. Intention-to-treat analysis therefore includes people who:

- Did not follow instructions
- Can no longer be located or contacted
- Withdrew from the trial
- Did not receive treatment

Including data from the groups above may weaken the results of a trial, but excluding the data would bias the trial. For instance, if half of the people in a treatment group withdrew because they thought the drug they were taking was ineffective and had severe side effects, and if the other half of the group had a 50 percent response rate, then excluding the data from the participants who withdrew makes the drug appear to be 50 percent effective. The actual response rate is 25 percent. Intention-to-treat analysis typically excludes participants who were ineligible to be included in the trial but were randomized.

Refer to the case study in section 7, page 73, for a review and summary of content covered in this workbook.

3
Advancing Cancer Care Through Clinical Trials

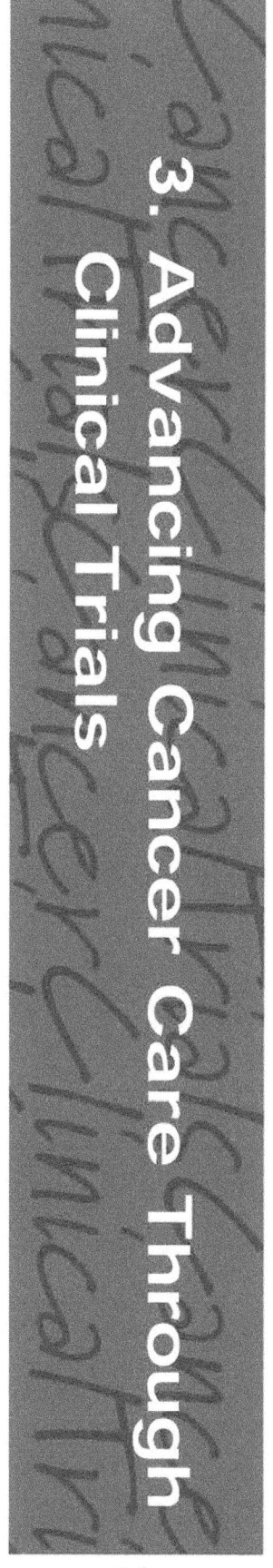

Learning Objectives
- Describe the FDA drug approval process
- Describe how clinical trial results are released
- Describe clinical trials that have led to advances in cancer prevention, detection, and treatment
- Discuss the importance of professional referral and patient participation in the research process

Once phase 1 and 2 treatment trials are completed, the data are analyzed and, if the treatment shows promise, it moves into phase 3 trials. As soon as the treatment sponsor thinks that phase 3 data show it is safe and superior to standard treatment, the sponsor may submit a New Drug Application (NDA) or a Biologics License Application (BLA), to FDA for approval. At this stage, FDA approves only the claim being made about the drug or intervention, not the drug or intervention itself.

FDA Approval Requirements

A New Drug Application includes:
- The exact chemical or biological makeup of the therapy and the mechanisms by which it is thought to be effective
- Results of animal studies
- Results of clinical trials
- How the drug or therapy is manufactured, processed, and packaged
- Quality control standards
- Information about drug or intervention samples of the product in the form(s) in which it is to be administered

FDA assesses applications in order of importance, giving first priority to interventions with the greatest potential benefits. All drugs that offer significant medical advances are considered priority drugs in the approval process.

Independent advisory committees of professionals from outside the agency give expert advice and guidance in making decisions about drug approval. By law, these committees include both a patient representative and a consumer representative. One such committee is the Oncologic Drugs Advisory Committee, which meets regularly to consider most cancer-related treatments and preventive drugs. The committee assesses the safety, effectiveness, and appropriate use of products considered for approval.

As FDA looks at the sponsor's data and its own review results, it applies two questions to each application:

1. Do the results of well-controlled clinical trials provide substantial evidence of effectiveness?
2. Do the results show that the product is safe under the proposed conditions of use? (In this context, "safe" means that potential benefits outweigh any known risks.)

Once FDA has approved a new drug, the drug is "labeled" for a specific use. This label includes information on eligibility, dose, safety, and adverse effects. The agency's responsibility for new treatments does not stop with final approval. FDA also:

- Implements and tracks programs to make sure manfacturers comply with standards and practice regulations
- Monitors new drug advertising to make sure it is truthful and complete
- Handles feedback from health professionals and consumers about effectiveness, adverse reactions, and potential problems in labeling and dosage

Releasing the Results

The results of a clinical trial are usually reported first in peer-reviewed scientific journals. If the results appear to have significant medical importance, researchers make a public announcement when the formal report is submitted for publication, ensuring that people benefit from the new treatment as soon as possible. Particularly important results are featured by the media and widely discussed at scientific meetings and within advocacy groups.

Clinical trial results are not available to the public as the trial progresses because:

- Knowing interim results could influence medical personnel and participants in the trial, biasing the results
- Statistical analysis might be less meaningful, compromising the accuracy of the findings

In the absence of very clear evidence that a trial should be stopped early for medical reasons, trials are completed before reporting results. Interim results are unavailable to the public, and often to the research teams. Independent data and safety monitoring boards track phase 3 trial data. These boards alert researchers about any safety or effectiveness issues that arise during the trial. Data and safety monitoring plans are also in place for many phase 1 and 2 trials.

Research progresses in small steps, and sometimes publishing the results of a trial is not as important as taking what was learned from the trial and building on it in a new trial. To find the results of a clinical trial, search a medical literature database, like Medline or PubMed, available online through the National Library of Medicine (*www.nlm.nih.gov*) and at medical institutions' libraries. The "closed protocol" file in NCI's PDQ® (Physician Data Query) may contain related studies (see section 6 for more information on PDQ).

It often takes more than a year for a scientific paper to be written, submitted, reviewed, edited, and published. If an initial literature search turns up nothing, try again after some time has passed.

Improving Cancer Care

Once an intervention is proven safe and effective, it may become the new standard of care. Thus, current cancer care is based on the results of past clinical trials. Recent clinical trials have resulted in the following treatment benefits for people with chronic myelogenous leukemia, cervical cancer, breast cancer, and melanoma.

Chronic Myelogenous Leukemia—A New Treatment Option

In 2001, FDA approved Gleevec™, offering a new treatment option for many people with chronic myelogenous leukemia (CML). Until then, bone marrow transplantation in the initial chronic phase of the disease was the only known effective therapy for CML. However, this is not an option for many people, and the procedure can cause serious side effects or death. Another option, treatment with the drug interferon alfa, may produce remission (a decrease in or disappearance of signs and symptoms of cancer) for many people. But if the drug is ineffective or people stop responding to it, their prognosis is generally bleak.

In three short-duration, early-phase clinical trials with Gleevec, researchers found that people with CML either had higher remission rates than expected or they had few side effects. Gleevec was designed to target an abnormal version of a cellular protein present in nearly all people with CML. The abnormal protein is much more active than the normal version and probably causes the disease. By blocking the abnormal protein, called BCR-ABL, Gleevec kills the leukemia cells.

Gleevec represents a new class of cancer drugs, which target abnormal proteins that are fundamental to the cancer itself.

Cervical Cancer—Improved Survival Rates

For many years, the standard therapy for invasive cervical cancer was surgery or radiation alone. Five large clinical trials showed that women with invasive cervical cancer have improved survival rates when they receive a cisplatin-containing chemotherapy regimen plus radiation therapy.

Breast Cancer

Less Extensive Surgery, Same Survival Time

For many years, the standard therapy for all breast cancers was a modified radical mastectomy with radiation or chemotherapy. Clinical trials showed that for women with early-stage disease, long-term survival after lumpectomy with axillary lymph node dissection plus radiation therapy is similar to survival after modified radical mastectomy.

Reduced Risk for Women at High Risk

Traditionally, women seeking to reduce their risk of breast cancer had no clear option. A large phase 3 clinical trial assessed risk reduction in women taking the drug tamoxifen. The trial found that high-risk women who took the drug for up to 5 years (an average of 4 years) had 49 percent fewer diagnoses of invasive breast cancer than those taking a placebo.

Melanoma—Improved Survival

According to the findings of a large, randomized clinical trial, compared with low-dose interferon or no therapy, high-dose interferon alfa-2b (Intron-A) significantly prolongs disease-free survival for people at high risk for melanoma recurrence.

Biological Therapy

Biological therapy (sometimes called immunotherapy, biotherapy, or biological response modifier therapy) uses the body's immune system, either directly or indirectly, to fight cancer or to lessen the side effects that some cancer treatments might cause.

The immune system is a complex network of cells and organs that work together to defend the body against attacks by "foreign," or "nonself," invaders. This network is one of the body's main defenses against disease. It works against disease, including cancer, in a variety of ways. For example, the immune system may recognize the difference between healthy cells and cancer cells in the body, and work to eliminate those that become cancerous.

Biological therapies are designed to repair, stimulate, or enhance the immune system's responses. Many clinical trials are testing the use of biological therapies, such as monoclonal antibodies and vaccines, to treat cancer.

Monoclonal Antibodies

Monoclonal antibodies (MOABs) are a form of biological therapy now being studied in the laboratory and in clinical trials.

MOABs are designed to fill a critical gap in the body's immune system. Although the human body naturally produces antibodies to identify and fight off viral and bacterial infections, the immune system may not always recognize cancer cells as harmful. This is because some cancer cells do not possess an antigen on their cell membrane that is capable of eliciting an immune response. Therefore, cancer is able to grow and spread unchecked. MOABs are being developed to supplement the body's immune system by recognizing and attacking specific proteins that cancer cells express. These specific antibodies may be active on their own, or they may be linked to a drug to allow specific delivery of the drug to the cancer cell.

Basic immunologic research identified a molecule specific to the surface of B-lymphocytes that also is highly expressed on the surface of most lymphomas. An antibody directed against this molecule was shown to be capable of killing cells. Over several years, researchers tried to engineer the antibody and succeeded. In 1997 FDA approved rituximab, now used to treat people with low-grade lymphoma.

Cancer Vaccines

Cancer vaccines are another form of biological therapy being studied in the laboratory and in clinical trials. Researchers are developing vaccines that may promote the recognition of cancer cells by a person's immune system. These vaccines may help the body reject tumors and prevent cancer from recurring. In contrast to vaccines against infectious diseases, cancer vaccines are designed to be injected after the disease is diagnosed, rather than before it develops. Vaccines given when the tumor is small may be able to eradicate the cancer. Cancer vaccines being tested in clinical trials are designed to treat cancer by getting the immune system to attack existing cancerous cells. Many vaccines are not used alone, but in combination with surgery, chemotherapy, or other interventions that help stimulate the immune response in general.

Early attempts to vaccinate people with cancer against the disease have been directed largely at melanoma, a potentially deadly skin cancer with easily accessible tumors. Researchers are also conducting studies that may lead to the development of vaccines for lymphoma, prostate, lung, breast, colon, and other cancers.

Speeding Up Drug Development

In the recent past, it has taken 15 years, on average, for an experimental drug to travel from the laboratory to U.S. consumers. Often the longest part of the process is finding people to participate in each clinical trial phase. With increased public awareness about clinical trials, more people may be willing to participate, and more professionals may refer people into appropriate trials. This awareness would ultimately reduce the time it takes for researchers to enroll participants in trials and complete them—and speed up the movement of new drugs or treatments into standard care.

Decisions to Advance Drug Development

Investigators make decisions about how to proceed with further research based on scientific evidence and promising basic research leads. Even if some participants in a clinical trial had a positive response to a new treatment, researchers must look at the global experience of all participants when deciding whether or not to continue or expand trials. In some trials, more participants treated with standard therapy may have better results than those treated with the experimental therapy, and the investigator may decide to continue research in a different direction.

The Drug Development and Approval Process

	Preclinical Testing		Clinical Trials			Post-Clinical Trials		Total Years for Drug Approval
	Step 1 Laboratory/ preclinical testing	Step 2 File IND[1] application with FDA[2]	Step 3 Phase 1	Step 4 Phase 2	Step 5 Phase 3	Step 6 File NDA[3] or BLA[4] with FDA	Step 7 FDA approval	
Purpose	Assess safety and biological activity in the laboratory and in animal models	Obtain FDA approval to begin clinical testing in humans after promising results in laboratory	Determine what dosage is safe, how treatment should be given	Evaluate effective-ness, look for side effects	Determine whether the new treatment (or new use of a treatment) is a better alternative to current standard	Inform the FDA of Phase 3 data which supports drug safety and better performance over current standard treatment	Review process/ approval	
All anticancer drugs (average number of years)	4.4 years		8.6 years				1.4 years	14.4 years
All drugs* (average number of years)	3.8 years		10.4 years				1.5 years	15.7 years

[1]IND = Investigational New Drug   [2]FDA = Food and Drug Administration
[3]NDA = New Drug Application   [4]BLA = Biologics License Application

* Classified as "new chemical entities," which exclude diagnostic agents, vaccines, and other biological compounds.
Sources: DiMasi, J.A. (2001). New drug development in the United States 1963-1999. *Clinical Pharmacology and Therapeutics*, May; 69(5); Tufts Center for the Study of Drugs Development, Tufts University; adapted from Pharmaceutical Research and Manufacturers of America.

Refer to the case study in section 7, page 73, for a review and summary of content covered in this workbook.

4
Participant Protection in Clinical Trials

Learning Objectives
- Recognize historical events and their influence on the development of safeguards for participants in clinical trials
- Identify Government regulations and agencies related to patient protection
- Describe current methods of participant protection that are implemented throughout the research process

Evolution of Participant Protection

The strong national and international safeguards in place today to protect research participants evolved from notorious abuses of human rights in the past. The first formal statement of medical ethics regarding research in humans emerged from the 1946 trial and conviction in Nuremberg, Germany, of Nazi physicians and scientists who conducted experiments on concentration camp inmates during World War II. The Nuremberg Code outlined broad concepts for the protection of human subjects and forms the basis of today's international code of ethics for the conduct of research.

In the United States, three infamous clinical trials called attention to the need for participant protection:

- *The Tuskegee syphilis study*, held from 1932 to 1972, followed—but did not treat—poor black men who had syphilis. During the trial, the men were offered "special free medical care" and were told that they would be treated for "bad blood." Instead, more than 400 men with syphilis and 200 men without the disease who served as controls were enrolled in an observational clinical trial without their knowledge or consent. By 1963, it was apparent that many more infected men than controls had developed complications, and 10 years later a report on the trial indicated that

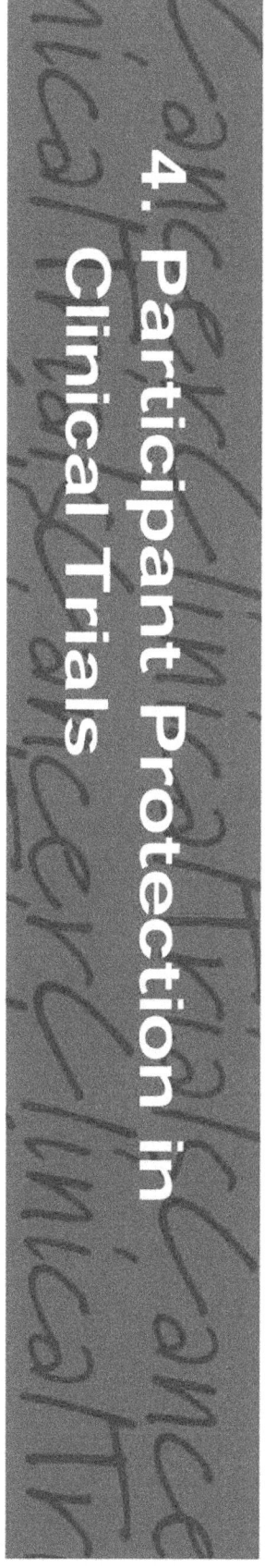

the death rate among those with syphilis was roughly double that of the controls. In the 1940s, penicillin was found to be effective in the treatment of syphilis, but researchers in the trial, which continued for almost 30 years after the discovery, neither informed nor treated subjects with the antibiotic.

- From 1963 to 1966, researchers deliberately infected newly admitted "mentally defective" children at the *Willowbrook School*, a State school in New York, with the hepatitis virus in order to study the natural history of the disease under controlled circumstances. In some cases, parents were not allowed to admit children to the institution unless they agreed to let them participate in the trials.

- In 1963, physician-investigators at the *Jewish Chronic Disease Hospital* in Brooklyn, New York, injected cancer cells grown in the lab into people hospitalized with various chronic diseases without informing the people or gaining their consent. In review proceedings, the Board of Regents of the State University of New York found that the trial had not been presented to the hospital's research committee; the researchers were found guilty of fraud, deceit, and unprofessional conduct.

In 1974, in response to these tragedies, the President established the National Commission for the Protection of Human Subjects of Biomedical and Behavioral Research. In 1979, the commission issued the Belmont Report, which delineated the ethical principles upon which today's regulations regarding research participants in the United States are based:

- **Respect for persons**—recognition of the personal dignity and autonomy of individuals, as well as special protections for people with diminished autonomy

- **Beneficence**—the obligation to protect people from harm by maximizing unanticipated benefits and minimizing possible risk of harm

- **Justice**—fairness in the distribution of research benefits and burdens

In addition, the commission concluded that "a permanent board with the authority to regulate at least all federally supported research involving human subjects" should be formed.

In response, Congress passed the National Research Act, which mandated the establishment of IRBs to review all U.S. Department of Health and Human Services (DHHS)-funded research. The procedures established for IRBs were further delineated and revised in 1981.

For more details on the history of participant protection, the role of the IRB, and patient confidentialy, see *http://cme.cancer.gov.*

Government Oversight

Two similar sets of regulations—enforced by HHS's Office for Human Research Protections (OHRP) and FDA—are in place to ensure the protection of clinical trial participants. If a trial is Government-supported and it involves an FDA-regulated drug or device, then it is subject to both sets of regulations. The basic requirements for IRBs and informed consent are congruent in the two sets of regulations.

Office for Human Research Protections

The Office for Human Research Protections (OHRP), formerly called the Office of Protection from Research Risks, safeguards participants in federally funded research and provides unity and leadership for 17 Federal departments and agencies that carry out research involving human participants. OHRP enforces an important regulation called the Common Rule (Title 45 CFR Part 46, Subpart A). The Common Rule sets standards for:
* Informed consent process
* Formation and function of IRBs
* Involvement of prisoners, children, and other vulnerable groups in research
* Many other protective measures

Researchers must provide written statements describing the

organization of the IRB, its procedures for approving trials, and how clinical trial participants are protected.

Although breaches in participant protection seldom occur, recent discoveries of inadequate protection have prompted the restatement of oversight goals and the addition of some new requirements by OHRP and the National Institutes of Health (NIH) to strengthen enforcement of the Common Rule, including:

- Aggressive efforts to improve the education and training of clinical research staff, IRB members, and staff research administrators regarding protection
- Guidelines to reaffirm the need to audit informed consent records for evidence of full compliance and confirmation of consent by investigators
- Submission of monitoring plans for all phase 1 and 2 clinical trials and the presence of a data and safety monitoring board for phase 3 trials
- Additional information to clarify regulations regarding conflict of interest

For a detailed proposal of the Government oversight goals set forth by former HHS Secretary Donna Shalala, see "Protecting Research Subjects—What Must Be Done" in the September 14, 2000, issue of the *New England Journal of Medicine (343: 808-810).*

Food and Drug Administration

FDA has its own regulations and policies on IRB review, informed consent, and participant protection (Title 21 CFR Parts 50 and 56). The regulations apply to any clinical trial that involves an investigational drug, biological product, or other device regulated by FDA, regardless of whether the trial receives Federal funding. FDA periodically inspects IRB records and operations to certify the adequacy of approvals, human subject safeguards, and the conduct of business.

Protecting Participants Before a Clinical Trial Begins

Scientific Review by Sponsor

Clinical trials that are sponsored by NCI are reviewed through different types of panels, including experts who review the scientific and technical merit of the proposed research. Many other clinical trial sponsors, such as pharmaceutical companies, also seek expert advice on the merits of their studies. Typical issues addressed by members of expert panels include:

- **Significance**: Does the trial address an important problem? If its aims are achieved, how will scientific knowledge be advanced? What effect will the trial have on current concepts or methods in the field?
- **Approach**: Are the conceptual framework, design, methods, and analyses adequately developed, well-integrated, and appropriate? Does the applicant acknowledge potential problem areas and consider alternative tactics?
- **Innovation**: Does the project employ novel concepts, approaches, or methods? Are the aims original and innovative? Does the project challenge existing paradigms or develop new methodologies or technologies?
- **Investigator**: Do the principal investigator and other researchers have sufficient training and experience to carry out the project?
- **Environment**: Does the scientific environment in which the work will be done contribute to the probability of success? Do the proposed experiments take advantage of unique features of the scientific environment or employ useful collaborative arrangements? Is there evidence of institutional support?

Institutional Review Board (IRB) Approval

An IRB functions as both a clearinghouse and a monitor of clinical trials. It determines whether the risks involved in a clinical trial are reasonable with respect to the potential benefits, and it must approve any clinical trial before it begins. The IRB also monitors the ongoing progress of the research.

Federal regulations require that an IRB include at least five people from diverse occupations and backgrounds. In addition, one member must be outside the sponsoring institution—that is, not connected to it by employment or relatives. To meet these requirements, IRBs are usually made up of a mix of medical specialists, nurses, other health care professionals, ethicists, and lay members from the community.

Most institutions that carry out clinical trials have their own review boards (there are roughly 3,000 IRBs in the United States). In some cases, a small institution might arrange for its research to be reviewed by another IRB rather than set up its own. All trials that are federally funded or evaluate a new drug or medical device regulated by FDA must be submitted to an IRB. However, many institutions require that all clinical trials conducted in their facilities, regardless of funding source, be IRB-approved. Before a trial can begin, the principal investigator submits an application to an IRB. The board reviews it on the basis of the following criteria:

- Risks to participants are minimized as much as possible through sound research design
- Risks to participants are reasonable in relation to the anticipated benefits and the knowledge that may result
- Participant selection is equitable
- Informed consent is sought in accordance with 45 CFR Part 46.116
- Informed consent is documented in accordance with 45 CFR Part 46.116
- Provisions are made for monitoring the data collected to ensure the safety of participants
- Provisions are made to protect the privacy of participants and the confidentiality of data collected during the trial
- Additional safeguards are in place if any participants are likely to be vulnerable to coercion or undue influence (e.g., children, prisoners, people with mental disabilities, or people with low income or education levels)

The IRB decides whether to approve the clinical trial and notifies the researcher and the institution in writing. The IRB may specify changes the researcher must make in order to gain approval.

After approving a trial, the IRB must decide how frequently to monitor it—usually on the basis of the risk involved. At the very least, the trial's progress must be reviewed yearly.

Informed Consent

Informed consent, as a legal, regulatory, and ethical concept, is an integral part of research. In clinical trials, informed consent is the process of providing all relevant information about the trial's purpose, risks, benefits, alternatives, and procedures to a potential participant, who then, consistent with his or her own interests and circumstances, makes an informed decision about whether or not to participate. Before agreeing to take part in a clinical trial, participants have the right to:

- Learn everything that is involved in the trial—including all details about treatment, tests, and possible risks and benefits
- Both hear and read the information in language they can understand

Informed Consent Documents

The informed consent *form* or *document* provides a summary of the clinical trial and explains a participant's rights. It is designed to begin the informed consent *process*. The participant acknowledges that he or she is entering a study, has been told what it involves, and understands the potential risks and benefits of participating.

Although reputable researchers do not try to fool people or sign them up against their will, individuals sometimes have difficulty understanding the information about a trial before agreeing to participate. Individuals may not understand the medical terminology and/or clinical requirements of a study, and they should be encouraged to ask questions until they understand all aspects of treatment. For many people it is important to ask a friend or family member to come with them when they receive information about medical options to be sure all important questions are raised. Some people may want to take notes or bring a tape recorder to assist them with questions and recall.

The following elements of informed consent are required under the Common Rule (Title 45 CFR Part 46, Subpart A):

- Statement that the trial involves research
- Explanation and description of the nature of the trial, purpose of the trial, duration of participation, procedures to be followed, and which procedures are experimental
- Description of foreseeable risks and discomforts
- Benefits to the participant and others
- Alternative procedures or treatments
- Description of the confidentiality of records
- Explanation of procedures if the project involves more than minimal risk (e.g., compensation, availability of medical treatment)
- Contact person for questions
- Statement that participation is voluntary, that there will be no loss of benefits on withdrawal, and that the participant may withdraw at any time
- Statement that the participant's signature indicates a decision to participate, having read and discussed the information presented

Any research trial, regardless of whether it is federally funded, should provide this information to participants in an informed consent document.

NCI has issued recommendations designed to help research institutions and clinical centers write comprehensive, user-friendly informed consent documents. Its Working Group on Informed Consent also developed a template and sample forms that serve as models for covering all of the information that Federal regulations require. To view the template or other documents related to informed consent, see the clinical trials section of *www.cancer.gov*.

Pediatric Assent to Participate

Children and adolescents are not deemed capable of giving true informed consent, so they are asked for their assent to (or dissent from) participation in a clinical trial. The trial must be explained in age-appropriate language or using visual aids. Parents or guardians are asked to give informed permission for their child to participate in a trial.

Assent must be obtained from all children and young people over age 7 unless:

- The child is found to be incapable of assenting
- The clinical trial offers a treatment or procedure that "holds out a prospect of direct benefit that is important to the health or well-being of the child and is available only in the context of the research" (in other words, if the trial offers a treatment that is thought to be better than those currently available or if it offers the only alternative to those available)

Even in these cases, permission from the parent or guardian is required. For more information, see the clinical trials section of *www.cancer.gov*.

Protecting Participants During a Clinical Trial

Informed Consent Process

The informed consent *process* provides people with ongoing explanations that will help them make educated decisions about whether to begin or to continue participation in a clinical trial. The process does not end with the signing of informed consent documents. If new benefits, risks, or side effects are discovered during the trial, researchers must inform participants. Participants are encouraged to ask questions at any time.

Institutional Review Board Role

During the initial review process, the IRB establishes how often a clinical trial should be monitored. Monitoring occurs at least yearly but sometimes more frequently. During these review sessions, the IRB examines a progress report provided by the clinical researcher in charge of the project. The report describes:

- How many people are enrolled in the trial
- How many have withdrawn
- Participants' experiences, including benefits and adverse effects
- Progress to date

Based on this information, the IRB decides whether the project should continue as described in the original research plan and, if not, what changes need to be made. An IRB can decide to suspend or terminate approval of a clinical trial if the researcher is not following requirements or if the trial appears to be causing serious harm to participants.

Data and Safety Monitoring Board (DSMB) Role

NIH requires that all phase 3 clinical trials undergo monitoring by a DSMB, and that all phase 1 and 2 clinical trials have a data and safety monitoring plan. A DSMB may also be appropriate and necessary for phase 1 and 2 clinical trials that are blinded, take place at multiple clinical sites, or employ particularly high-risk interventions or vulnerable populations.

The DSMB is an independent committee whose membership includes, at a minimum, a statistician and a clinical expert in the area being studied. Other members are experts in all scientific disciplines needed to interpret the data and ensure participant safety. Members may also be clinical trial experts, statisticians, bioethicists, or other clinicians knowledgeable about the trial's subject matter.

The objectives of data and safety monitoring plans are to:
• Ensure that risks associated with participation are minimized to the extent practical and possible
• Ensure the integrity of data
• Stop a trial if safety concerns arise or if its objectives are met

Ending Trials Early

There can be compelling reasons for halting a trial early. If participants experience severe side effects, or if there is clear evidence that risks outweigh benefits, the IRB and DSMB will recommend that the trial be stopped early. A trial might also be stopped if there is clear evidence that the new intervention is effective—in order to make it widely available.

Breast Cancer Prevention Trial

The Breast Cancer Prevention Trial, conducted by NCI's National Surgical Adjuvant Breast and Bowel Project, was designed to evaluate whether taking the drug tamoxifen could prevent breast cancer in women considered to be at high risk of developing the disease. In March 1998, interim data showed that tamoxifen cut the chance of getting breast cancer almost in half. Instead of continuing the trial for the full 5 years, as planned, researchers stopped the trial after about 4 years.

Women in the trial who were taking tamoxifen were offered the opportunity to continue treatment for the remaining 14 months of the trial. Women receiving the placebo were invited to participate in the Study of Tamoxifen and Raloxifene, or STAR trial, designed to determine whether the osteoporosis prevention drug raloxifene is as effective as tamoxifen in reducing the chance of developing breast cancer. The women's other option was to seek tamoxifen from a physician on their own, outside a clinical trial.

B-14 Trial

Another trial involving tamoxifen and conducted by the National Surgical Adjuvant Breast and Bowel Project, the B-14 trial, was also halted early—but for a different reason. This trial, which started in 1982, enrolled women who had had surgery for cancer that was limited to the breast. After surgery, the women took either tamoxifen or a placebo for 5 years to determine whether tamoxifen would prevent recurrence of the cancer. Five years into the trial, significantly more of the women taking tamoxifen remained disease-free, so the trial was extended another 5 years. Women who had been taking tamoxifen were given the opportunity to reenroll in the trial and be randomly assigned to take tamoxifen or placebo for an additional 5 years.

The extended trial was cut short when several interim data analyses showed that the tamoxifen group had a slightly higher rate of cancer recurrence than the placebo group. Statistical analysis showed that no additional benefit was to be gained by continuing tamoxifen for more than 5 years. The trial was halted, and the women stopped taking tamoxifen beyond 5 years.

Before taking part in any clinical trial, health care professionals and their patients should make sure it is reputable by getting answers to these important questions:
- What is the purpose of the study or therapy?
- Who has reviewed and approved it?
- What are the credentials of its researchers and personnel?
- What information or results is it based on?
- How are study data and patient safety being monitored?
- How will the results be shared?

Quality Assurance Monitoring

NCI has several ways of ensuring the quality of data collected during clinical trials. Many trials, for example, have committees that review major elements of the study for accuracy, such as:
- Pathology
- Radiotherapy
- Surgery
- Administration of investigational drugs

In addition, data management and statistical centers use quality control measures to help identify and correct or clarify inconsistencies and inaccuracies in submitted data.

Another part of NCI's quality assurance program is onsite monitoring, or audits, of trial procedures, documents, and data. Institutions are audited at least once every 3 years. Auditors review three main areas:
1. Conformance to IRB and informed consent requirements
2. Shipping, storage, and use of drugs and other agents
3. Individual participants' cases

Adverse Event Reporting

An adverse event is any unanticipated problem involving risks to clinical trial participants or others. For more information on adverse event reporting, see the clinical trials section of the Web site *www.cancer.gov*.

Refer to the case study in section 7, page 73, for a review and summary of content covered in this workbook.

5
Barriers to Clinical Trial Participation

Learning Objectives
- Compare and contrast benefits and risks of participating in cancer clinical trials
- Identify barriers that deter health care professionals from referring patients to clinical trials
- Identify barriers for low participation in cancer clinical trials
- Identify barriers that deter special populations (ethnic minorities, people with limited proficiency in English, elderly persons) from participating in clinical trials
- Recognize cost and insurance issues related to participation in clinical trials

A 1999 press release from the American Society of Clinical Oncologists revealed that only 3 percent of adults with cancer participate in clinical trials—far fewer than the number needed to answer the most pressing cancer questions quickly.

The reasons so few adults participate in clinical trials are complex and involve both participant and professional issues. Ideas to address these problems can be found in *Cancer Clinical Trials: A Resource Guide for Outreach, Education, and Advocacy*, also available from NCI.

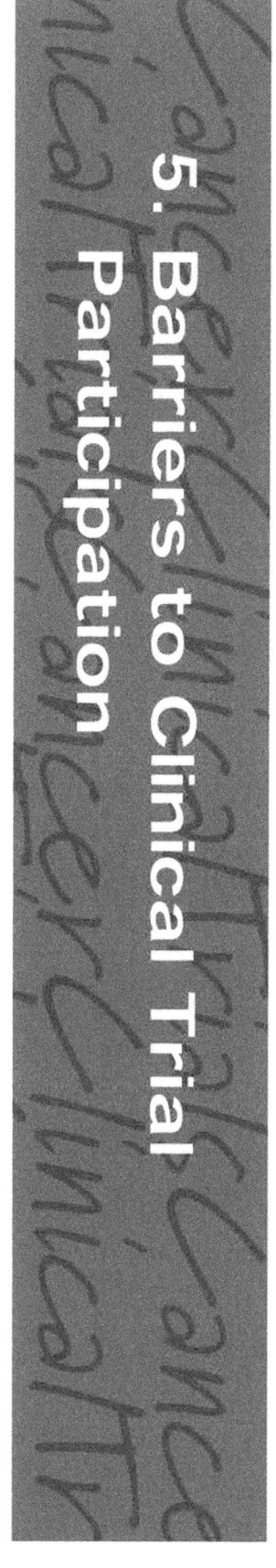

5. Barriers to Clinical Trial Participation

Barriers for Health Care Professionals

- **Lack of awareness of appropriate clinical trials.** Physicians are not always aware of available clinical trials. Some may not be aware of the local resources, or some may assume that none would be appropriate for their patients.
- **Unwillingness to "lose control" of a person's care.** Most doctors feel that the relationship they have with their patients is very important. They want what is best for the patient, and if the person must be referred elsewhere to participate in a trial, doctors fear they may lose control of the person's care.
- **Belief that standard therapy is best.** Many health care providers may not adequately understand how clinical trials are conducted or their importance. Some believe that the treatment in clinical trials is not as good as the standard treatment. They also might be uncomfortable admitting that there is uncertainty about which treatment is best in a phase 3 clinical trial.
- **Belief that referring and/or participating in a clinical trial adds an administrative burden.** The length and details of most research protocols may deter providers from participating in clinical trials. The possibility of incurring additional costs and expenses that might be inadequately reimbursed is a deterrent for many.
- **Concerns about the person's care or how the person will react to the suggestion of clinical trial participation.**

Strategies for Addressing Barriers

- Provide checklists on patient charts with eligibility criteria, placing posters with open protocols listed, or using abridged "protocol pocket cards" with key inclusion and exclusion criteria.
- Dedicate one research nurse or research assistant to identifying and screening participants, coordinating pre-enrollment tests, educating participants about the protocol and process, and initiating the informed consent and enrollment process.
- Access funding for clinical trial support. See the *www.cancer.gov* site section on clinical trials, the CTSU site (*www.ctsu.org*), and the NCI Cooperative Group sites for information.

Barriers for the General Population

- **Lack of awareness of clinical trials.** Research has consistently shown that most people with cancer are not aware of the option to participate in clinical trials.
- **Lack of access to trials.** The reality or the perception that there are no trials nearby deters many potential participants. In addition, seeking care at a distant trial site presents time and travel barriers.
- **Fear, distrust, or suspicions of research.** For many people, the loss of control (not choosing their treatment) that comes with entering a randomized trial is too great. Many also fear being treated like "guinea pigs" or being "experimented upon," as well as not receiving treatment for their cancer. People may have a general lack of trust in the medical profession based on past negative experiences or the knowledge of historical abuses of research participants.
- **Practical or personal obstacles.** Costs of being away from work and family may be deterrents for some people. Others may not wish to leave the care of their own physician. People from certain racial or ethnic groups or who are medically underserved may feel that care within a trial will not be sensitive to their needs. Others may feel that recruitment strategies are not sensitive to their needs. Still others may believe that standard care is better than the treatment available in a trial.
- **Insurance or cost problems.** Another deterrent is the fear of being denied insurance coverage for participation in a clinical trial. If a person is uninsured, the cost of trial participation is an issue.
- **Unwillingness to go against personal physician's wishes.**

A Survey on Clinical Trial Barriers

A survey of almost 6,000 people with cancer conducted in 2000 took a look at why so few adults participate in cancer clinical trials. Some of the highlights included:

- About 85 percent of people with cancer were either unaware or unsure that participation in clinical trials was an option, though about 75 percent of these people said they would have been willing to enroll had they known it was possible.
- Of those who were aware of the clinical trial option, most declined to participate because they believed common myths about clinical trials. They either thought that:
  - The medical treatment they would receive in a clinical trial would be less effective than standard care
  - They might get a placebo
  - They would be treated like a "guinea pig"
  - Their insurance company would not cover costs
- People who received treatment through a clinical trial found it to be a very positive experience:
  - Ninety-seven percent said they were treated with dignity and respect and that the quality of care they received was "excellent" or "good"
  - Eighty-six percent said their treatment was covered by insurance

Source: Harris Interactive. *Health Care News* 1(3) [Poll]. (Available from *www.harrisinteractive.com/about/healthnews/ HI_HealthCareNews2001Vol1_iss3.pdf*)

Supported by the Coalition of National Cancer Cooperative Groups, the Cancer Research Foundation of America, the Cancer Leadership Council, and the Oncology Nursing Society.

Barriers for Diverse Populations

Additional barriers exist for people who are from certain ethnic/racial backgrounds or who are medically underserved. The following is not meant to be a comprehensive overview of all barriers associated with clinical trials, and what is outlined should not be generalized to all diverse populations.

Diverse U.S. Populations—Definitions

Diverse populations include minority ethnic and racial groups designated by the U.S. Government, including:

- American Indian or Alaska Native
- Asian American
- Black or African American
- Hispanic or Latin American
- Native Hawaiian or other Pacific Islander

Ethnically diverse populations are growing rapidly; in the 2000 Census, about 25 percent of the U.S. population reported their race as something other than White.

The National Cancer Institute's working definition of diverse populations also includes medically underserved populations. Medically underserved populations are those that lack easy access to, or don't make use of, high-quality cancer prevention, screening and early detection, treatment, or rehabilitation services. These may include people of any racial or ethnic group who live in rural areas, or who have low income or literacy levels. Medically underserved groups are generally characterized as experiencing higher cancer mortality rates and insufficient participation rates in cancer control programs.

Specific Barriers

- **Long-standing fear, apprehension, and skepticism** exist among some minority populations about medical research because of abuses that have happened in the past (e.g., the legacy of the Tuskegee syphilis study). Among these populations, there is often widespread fear and distrust of the medical care system as a result of discrimination, indifference, and disrespect. Many feel that they do not want to give up rights or lose power in order to be "experimented on." Others may be skeptical about the quality of care that would be provided in a clinical trial. Some may find that trial recruitment strategies are not sensitive to their needs.

- **Doctors may not mention clinical trials as an option** for cancer care. As noted above, many physicians do not refer people to clinical trials. Some physicians may avoid suggesting a clinical trial to people who belong to racial or ethnic minorities out of concern that people would see them as insensitive. Moreover, some physicians may inadvertently discriminate against older people or those from certain ethnic or cultural backgrounds.

- **People from various cultural or ethnic backgrounds hold different values and beliefs that may be different than principles of Western medicine.** Many people have cultural beliefs that Western medicine cannot address their health concerns. Different ethnic and cultural views of health and disease (e.g., fatalism, family decisions about treatment, use of "traditional healers," prayer, herbal medicines, or use of complementary/alternative health practices) may make clinical trials a less attractive treatment option. For prevention trials, many may feel that the risk of a potential disease and its consequences may be less important than meeting daily needs.

- **Language or literacy barriers** may make it difficult for some people to understand and consider participating. The complexity of forms, including informed consent documents, may also be a barrier to those considering participation. Translation can also be difficult if the person translating information has not had specialized training.

- **Additional access problems** confront many people. Depending on where they live or their access to transportation, people may have difficulty getting to a clinical trial site. Those with low incomes may find it difficult to take time off work or find appropriate childcare. Other barriers, such as a lack of health insurance or a source of health care, clearly present difficulties in accessing trials.

For some solutions to barriers for diverse populations, see NCI's *Cancer Clinical Trials: A Resource Guide for Advocacy, Education, and Outreach.*

Cost Barriers

The costs associated with clinical trials can be a barrier for many professionals and the public. Physicians are often concerned about reimbursement related to the expense of either caring for people enrolled in trials or offering trials within their practice. Potential trial participants often fear that their insurance company will not cover participation. Those who are uninsured will need to know how their participation in a trial will be covered.

There are two types of costs associated with clinical trials: participant care costs and research costs.

Participant Care Costs

Participant care costs include:

- **Usual care costs**, such as doctor visits, hospital stays, clinical laboratory tests, and x-rays, occur whether someone is participating in a trial or receiving standard treatment.
- **Extra care costs** are those associated with clinical trial participation, such as additional tests that may be required.

These costs may or may not be covered by a participant's health plan.

Research Costs

Research costs include costs associated with conducting the trial, such as:

- Data collection and management
- Research physician and nurse time
- Analysis of results
- Clinical laboratory tests and x-rays
- Cost of the agent being tested

Most of the time, research costs are covered by the sponsoring organization.

Health Plan Coverage

Health insurance companies and managed care plans do not always cover all care costs in a clinical trial. What they do cover varies by plan and by trial. Now that Medicare has developed a policy explicitly covering the routine care costs of diagnostic and treatment clinical trials, other insurers may follow suit.

Insurance companies often claim that paying for clinical trials would be too costly. But recent studies (Bennet et al., 2000; Fireman et al., 2000; Wagner et al., 1999) found that costs for participants in clinical trials are not appreciably higher than costs for people not enrolled in trials.

For coverage strategies for participants and professionals, see the clinical trials section of *www.cancer.gov*. Some insurance carriers that cover clinical trials will even help health care professionals locate appropriate trials.

Established vs. Investigational Therapies

In general, the most important factor determining coverage of a treatment is the health plan's judgment as to whether the therapy is "established" or "investigational." Health plans usually consider a treatment established if sufficient scientific data exist to show it is safe and effective. If a health plan does not think sufficient data exist, it may consider the service investigational. Thus, some health plans, especially smaller ones, will not cover any costs associated with a clinical trial. Policies vary widely, but in most cases it helps to have someone from the research team initiate discussions with the health plan.

Other Criteria

Health plans may specify other criteria a trial must meet in order to be covered, for example:

- **Sponsorship:** The trial must be sponsored by an organization whose review and oversight procedures meet the health plan's standards of scientific rigor.
- **Trial type and phase:** The trial must be judged "medically necessary" by the health plan; this determination is made on a case-by-case basis. In some cases, the trial must be in phase 3.

While a plan may be willing to cover costs associated with phase 3 trials, it may require documentation of known benefits before covering a phase 1 or 2 trial. Participants may have more difficulty getting coverage for costs associated with prevention and screening trials because health plans are currently less likely to have a review process in place for them.

- **Cost neutrality:** The trial must be cost-neutral—that is, it must not be significantly more expensive than treatments the health plan considers standard.
- **Lack of standard therapy:** The trial must offer treatment of a cancer for which no standard therapy is available.
- **Facility and personnel qualifications:** The facility and medical staff must meet specific health plan qualifications for conducting unusual services, especially intensive therapy such as a bone marrow transplant (high-dose chemotherapy with bone marrow/stem cell rescue).

Legislation and Policies

Despite interest at the Federal level, as of 2002, no legislation has been passed to require private health plans to uniformly cover all clinical trial costs. However, there have been several important developments at the Federal level regarding clinical trial coverage:

- Medicare reimburses for all routine participant care costs for its beneficiaries participating in clinical trials.
- Beneficiaries of TRICARE, the Department of Defense's health program, are covered for NCI-sponsored phase 2 and phase 3 prevention and treatment clinical trials.
- The Department of Veterans Affairs (VA) allows eligible veterans to participate in a broad range of NCI clinical trials across the country. The agreement covers all phases and types of NCI-sponsored trials.

Many States have also passed legislation or developed policies that require health plans to cover clinical trial costs. For an updated legislation listing, see the clinical trials section of the NCI Web site *www.cancer.gov*.

Refer to the case study in section 7, page 73, for a review and summary of content covered in this workbook.

6
Conducting, Referring to, and Locating Clinical Trials

Learning Objectives
- Describe the types of sponsorship of cancer clinical trials
- Define the role of the National Cancer Institute in conducting clinical trials throughout the United States
- Identify methods of referring patients to clinical trials
- Demonstrate ways of locating clinical trial resources

Sponsorship

In order to find a clinical trial, it is helpful to understand who sponsors trials. Clinical trials are sponsored by both Government and private organizations including the National Cancer Institute and pharmaceutical companies. Clinical trials take place all over the United States, in locations as diverse as a rural community clinic or a cancer center in a large urban area.

National Cancer Institute
NCI sponsors hundreds of clinical trials around the country through six major programs, which are discussed below.

Clinical Trials Cooperative Group Program
The Clinical Trials Cooperative Group Program supports a large network of organizations that continually generate and conduct new clinical trials consistent with national priorities in cancer treatment research. Member organizations carry out large, randomized phase 3 trials, as well as phase 2 trials.

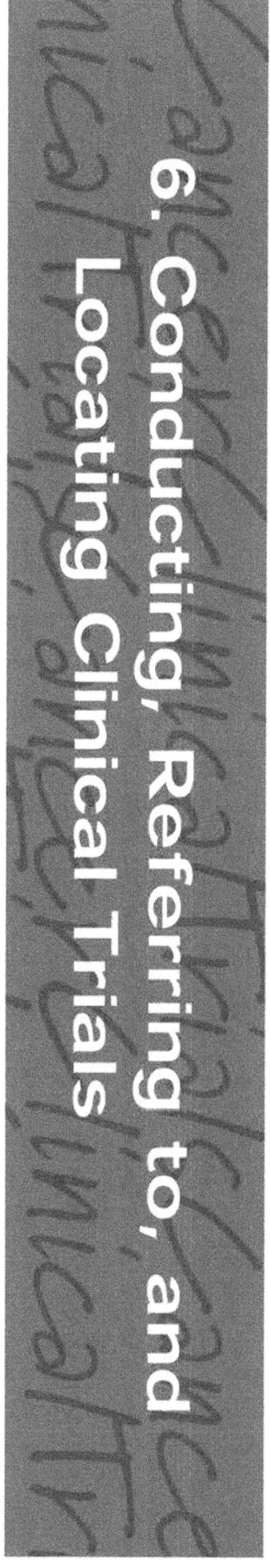

Members conduct clinical trials in locations nationwide, while administration and data are handled at a central location. Members of the groups include:

- Academic institutions
- NCI-designated cancer centers
- Physicians in the Community Clinical Oncology Program and the Minority-Based Community Clinical Oncology Program (described below)
- Community physicians and community hospitals

Each year, the groups enroll some 20,000 new people in treatment trials, evaluate some 12,000 new participants in ancillary studies, and follow the progress of many times that many participants in ongoing trials. Thousands of individual investigators participate in these studies. The cooperative groups have been instrumental in developing both new standards of care for people with cancer and sophisticated clinical investigation techniques.

There are 12 groups in the Clinical Trials Cooperative Group Program:
1. American College of Surgeons Oncology Group (ACOSOG)
2. Cancer and Acute Leukemia Group B (CALGB)
3. Children's Cancer Study Group (CCSG)
4. Eastern Cooperative Oncology Group (ECOG)
5. Gynecologic Oncology Group (GOG)
6. Intergroup Rhabdomyosarcoma Study Group (IRSG)
7. National Surgical Adjuvant Breast and Bowel Project (NSABP)
8. National Wilms Tumor Study Group (NWTSG)
9. North Central Cancer Treatment Group (NCCTG)
10. Pediatric Oncology Group (POG)
11. Radiation Therapy Oncology Group (RTOG)
12. Southwest Oncology Group (SWOG)

For more cooperative group information, see *http://ctep.info.nih.gov.*

Cancer Trials Support Unit

NCI and the Clinical Trials Cooperative Group Program are collaborating in a pilot project—the Cancer Trials Support Unit (CTSU)—to reduce administrative burdens and recruit more physicians to become involved in clinical trials.

CTSU is designed to streamline and centralize many administrative, financial, and data collection tasks. CTSU will provide participating physicians with a single access point to NCI's entire phase 3 clinical trial system, facilitating access to protocols, training, and educational information. Highlights of the fully developed system will include:

- Cross-group registration enabling physicians to register people on adult cooperative group trials in leukemia, lung, genitourinary, colorectal, and breast cancers, even if they are not members of the group conducting the trial
- Online registration, eligibility assessment, and reporting of data that will use a common format and state-of-the-art data management systems
- A coordinated auditing system that will eliminate multiple quality assurance audits for research personnel participating in more than one cooperative group
- Centralization of administrative tasks, including credentialing and verification of IRB approval for all investigators participating in cooperative groups and CTSU

CTSU opened in July 2000 for cooperative group members. If the initial experience is successful, oncologists not affiliated with a group will be encouraged to participate as well.

For more information about CTSU, see *www.ctsu.org.*

Community Clinical Oncology Program

The Community Clinical Oncology Program (CCOP) enables community physicians to work with investigators conducting NCI-supported clinical trials. The program increases the number of participants and physicians who can take part in clinical trials operated simultaneously in major research centers and in the community. It benefits investigators by giving them an opportunity to conduct large-scale cancer prevention and control studies at the community level.

Facilities participating in the program must be affiliated with an NCI-supported clinical cooperative group or cancer center and use research protocols developed by these groups.

Minority-Based Community Clinical Oncology Program

The Minority-Based Community Clinical Oncology Program (MBCCOP) was initiated in 1990 to provide people with cancer who belong to minority groups access to state-of-the-art treatment, prevention, and control technology. The minority-based program was begun because 40 percent of the people with cancer referred to CCOP physicians each year are from a minority group. Each MBCCOP pledges to accrue more participants from minority groups than other CCOPs do.

Since funding began, participant enrollment in the minority-based program has grown to account for approximately 10 percent of all ethnic minorities enrolled in NCI-approved clinical trials.

Cancer Centers Program

The Cancer Centers Program consists of more than 50 NCI-supported research centers. Each cancer center also belongs to at least one cooperative group.

NCI supports three types of centers:
1. **Comprehensive cancer centers**, which conduct basic, clinical, and preventive research programs, as well as community outreach and education programs
2. **Clinical cancer centers**, which conduct primarily clinical research programs but may have programs in other research areas as well
3. **Cancer centers** (formerly called Basic Science Cancer Centers), which conduct basic or preventive research programs and do not have clinical programs

Please refer to *http://cancer.gov/cancercenters* for a comprehensive list of cancer centers.

Clinical Grants Program

The Clinical Grants Program supports clinical researchers through various types of grants, all of which are peer reviewed.

Pharmaceutical and Biotech Companies

Pharmaceutical and biotech companies also conduct clinical trials, both locally and nationally. They may conduct these trials in collaboration with universities, hospitals, NCI, and local physicians. These trials are subject to the companies' own review panels and to an IRB, which may be local or national in scope.

Making Referrals

When a person is first diagnosed with cancer, his or her physician may suggest several possible options for treatment, possibly including a clinical trial. Likewise, a person at high risk of developing cancer may be offered prevention options that include a clinical trial.

Decisions concerning eligibility for cancer clinical trials are often complicated, requiring very specific information regarding a person's medical condition and prior treatment. For that reason, it is preferable to have a provider who is familiar with the person's case make the initial contact with clinical trial staff. A person who calls a researcher directly may have insufficient medical information, thereby making a decision about eligibility difficult and frustrating for both the potential participant and the researcher. Once contact is made, a referral coordinator may accept telephone, mail, or e-mail inquiries from physicians, potential participants, and others about the availability of clinical trials. Preliminary eligibility can be evaluated over the phone, and appointments with the clinical trial team can be scheduled if the person decides to proceed.

The informed consent process begins as soon as a potential participant begins to explore the trial with the clinical research team. The research team discusses the trial's purpose, procedures, risks, potential benefits, and participants' rights. After this dialogue, the person may wish to speak to his or her referring provider to review the information and help determine the best course.

If the person opts to enter the trial, the research team should send the referring provider relevant updates and followup information until the person returns to the provider's care.

Deciding to refer a person to a clinical trial is easier if the health care professional has adequate information regarding the trial's objectives and eligibility criteria. Before discussing a trial as an option, the professional should learn as much as possible about the trial.

Discussing Clinical Trials with Patients

Health care professionals may be able to assist potential trial participants in their decision by considering the following benefits and risks to clinical trial participation with their patients.

Possible Benefits of Clinical Trial Participation

- Participants will receive, at a minimum, the best standard treatment. This may be as good as, or better than, the new approach being tested.
- If a participant is taking the new treatment and it is shown to work, he or she may be among the first to benefit.
- By examining the benefits and drawbacks of clinical trials and other treatment choices, participants are taking an active role in a decision that affects their health care and life.
- Some participants feel good about helping advance medical knowledge that will improve cancer care and help others.
- Even when they don't lead to new therapies, clinical trials often answer important questions and help move research forward.

Possible Risks of Clinical Trial Participation

- New treatments are not always better than standard care.
- New treatments may have unexpected side effects that are worse than those of standard treatment.
- Although a new treatment is beneficial, it may not work for every participant. Even standard treatments do not help everyone.
- If a participant receives standard treatment instead of the new treatment being tested, it may not be as effective as the new approach.

- Participants may have additional patient care costs that are not covered by the study sponsor or by their health insurance or managed care plan.
- Participants may have to incur the costs of travel, childcare, lost work hours, hotels, and meals.
- Participation in a clinical trial may require increased patient responsibility, such as going to more appointments or self-monitoring for side effects.

Cancer Information and Clinical Trial Resources

NCI Resources

NCI's Web site, *www.cancer.gov*, provides access to a wealth of information on clinical cancer care. The site contains information from PDQ® (Physician Data Query), including the latest information about cancer treatment, screening, prevention, genetics, supportive care, and complementary and alternative medicine, as well as a registry of cancer clinical trials. Clinical oncology specialists review current literature from more than 70 medical journals, evaluate its relevance, and synthesize it into clear summaries, which are then reviewed monthly and updated as needed based on new information. Most cancer information summaries appear in two versions: 1) a technical version for the health professional and 2) a nontechnical version for patients, their families, and the public. Many of the summaries are also available in Spanish.

The NCI Web site also includes approximately 100 fact sheets on various cancer-related topics, information on ordering NCI publications, and educational features and news summaries concerning the latest results from cancer clinical trials.

NCI also has a Web-based continuing education tutorial on implementing clinical trials into your practice. This tutorial provides information for health care professionals interested in referring patients to trials, and more detailed information for health care professionals interested in actually implementing clinical trials into their practice. The series is available at *http://cme.cancer.gov*.

The clinical trials registry PDQ contains more than 1,800 ongoing clinical trials, with information about trials around the world. All clinical trials undergo review prior to inclusion. Although no single resource lists every cancer clinical trial being conducted in the United States and abroad, PDQ is the most comprehensive cancer clinical trials registry, and contains information about trials sponsored by NCI, the pharmaceutical industry, and some international groups. Users can narrow their search by multiple parameters, such as stage of disease, phase of trial, treatment modality, and geographic location. PDQ also contains an archival file of more than 11,000 clinical trials that are no longer accepting participants, including contact information for principal investigators of trials that may not yet be published in the biomedical literature.

Accessing NCI's Clinical Trial and Cancer Information by Phone
NCI's Cancer Information Service—NCI's Cancer Information Service is a national information and education network for patients, the public, and health professionals. From regional offices covering the entire United States, Puerto Rico, and the U.S. Virgin Islands, trained staff provide the latest cancer information through a toll-free telephone service. Staff can respond to calls in either English or Spanish. The Cancer Information Service, with regional offices throughout the United States, may work with organizations and professionals to plan, implement, and evaluate culturally appropriate clinical trials education programs using the Clinical Trials Education Series.

> Access: The toll-free number is 1-800-4-CANCER (1-800-422-6237). For deaf and hard of hearing callers with TTY equipment, the number is 1-800-332-8615. Hours of operation are Monday through Friday, 9:00 a.m. to 4:30 p.m., local time. Callers also have the option of listening to recorded information about cancer 24 hours a day, 7 days a week.

NIH Web Site

No single resource lists every cancer clinical trial being conducted in the United States and abroad. However, in 2000 the National Institutes of Health launched a new Web site, *www.clinicaltrials.gov*, that aims to be a complete listing of all U.S. Government- and industry-sponsored clinical trials, including cancer trials.

The site contains approximately 7,200 clinical trials, most of them Government-sponsored. However, additional trials from the pharmaceutical industry are being added.

Other Web Sites

The Internet includes a variety of clinical trial databases and matching services. The owners of these sites can be:
- **Not-for-profit organizations,** that might:
  - Use volunteers to provide content
  - Be supported by an academic institution or foundation
- **For-profit organizations,** that might:
  - Receive a fee from pharmaceutical companies every time a person signs up for a trial
  - Give some of its profits back to the cancer community

Anyone interested in using online services to find a clinical trial should ask questions and evaluate the information before submitting personal information or calling an investigator from the service:
- Who owns/runs the site?
- Where does the financial backing come from?
- How does the service get paid? By matching people to trials? By clinical trial submission to the database? Other?
- Does anyone make money on this site? If so, who?
- What is the source of clinical trial information?
- Does the site include all clinical trials? All Government-supported trials? All pharmaceutical trials?

People may wish to look at information from many sites and consider the source of the information before making important health-related decisions.

Refer to the case study in section 7, page 73, for a review and summary of content covered in this workbook.

Guide To Finding Clinical Trial Resources

	What is it?	How do I access it?	What will it provide?
National Cancer Institute's PDQ	Database produced by NCI Registry of approximately 1,800 active cancer clinical trials	Go to **www.cancer.gov** Go to the clinical trials area and follow the search directions OR Call 1-800-4-CANCER	Summaries about clinical trials conducted by NCI-sponsored researchers, the pharmaceutical industry, and some international groups
National Library of Medicine	Database produced by NIH Registry now lists 4,000 primarily NIH-supported clinical studies on many conditions, and more will be added All trials on PDQ are listed in this database	Go to **www.clinicaltrials.gov** Can browse by disease or sponsor or insert key words	Summaries about clinical trials for a wide range of conditions—most of the trials listed are sponsored by NIH
Food and Drug Administration's Cancer Clinical Trials Directory	A list of sources prepared by FDA's Office of Special Health Issues Guides user to other Web locations for institutions that conduct or list cancer clinical trials	Go to **www.fda.gov/oashi/ cancer/trials.html#table** Can browse by disease for different sources	Web addresses and telephone numbers Information listed on the Web sites in this directory varies widely
Local Cancer Center Web Sites	Locally produced Web sites that include listings for trials sponsored by NCI and some pharmaceutical companies Good supplementary resources for locating clinical trials; a cancer center may begin participating in an NCI-sponsored trial before the center's information is listed in CancerNet/PDQ	Different sites can be found through: • **www.cancer.gov** • Local institutions • Call 1-800-4-CANCER for a center near you Information on trials taking place at NCI's Clinical Center in Bethesda, Maryland is available at **http://ccr.nci.nih.gov** then select "clinical trials" Some centers may also have telephone information centers	Information that varies from center to center
Examples of Pharmaceutical Resources/ Internet Clinical Trial Matching Sites	Pharmaceutical Research and Manufacturers of America (PhRMA) publishes a list of new cancer drugs in development CenterWatch's Clinical Trials Listing Service and Emerging Med.com's clinical trials matching service list many industry- and Government-sponsored trials	**PhRMA** Go to **http://www.phrma.org** Click on "New Medicines in Development" and search by disease. The drugs are listed by cancer type. Or call 202-835-3400. **CenterWatch** Go to **www.centerwatch.com** Click on "Trial Listings" and then "CenterWatch Trial Listings by Medical Areas" or call 617-856-5900. **EmergingMed.com** Go to **http://www.emergingmed.com**	Descriptions, sites, telephone numbers, and investigator names by State

7
Case Study

The Clinical Case

Mr. Joe Smith, a 59-year-old African American male, presents to his primary care physician, Dr. Bob Brown, in rural Wisconsin. He has been complaining of difficulty with initiating urination and frequency. He presents clinically with an abnormal rectal exam and an elevated prostate-specific antigen (PSA) of 8 ng/ml (normal in a 59-year-old Black male is less than 4 ng/ml). Mr. Smith's mass is biopsied and the results reveal a prostatic tumor. The nearest comprehensive cancer center is 100 miles away, and Mr. Smith wants to be treated by Dr. Brown. He says he wants to stay close to his home and family, and does not want to be cared for by "those big city doctors."

Mr. Smith decides to undergo a radical prostatectomy at his community hospital. Surgery reveals a 1.5 cm tumor with clear margins, negative pelvic node involvement, and unilateral seminal vesicle involvement, which puts Mr. Smith at high risk for eventual tumor spread. To complete his clinical staging, a bone scan and CT scan are completed. Mr. Smith's tumor is formally staged. At his 3-month followup visit, post-operatively, his PSA is 0.2 (undetectable).

Dr. Brown closely follows Mr. Smith. Three years after his surgery his PSA has slowly risen to 11, but his bone scan and CT scans remain negative. Dr. Brown informs Mr. Smith that there are many clinical trials for men with prostate cancer at all stages. He explains that these trials are being conducted to try to find the best methods for cancer prevention, early detection, and treatment. At this point in his disease, Mr. Smith does not wish to consider a clinical trial, so he continues to receive standard care. Dr. Brown recommends starting standard treatment with hormone therapy injections monthly. The patient's PSA drops to less than 0.2 again.

Two years later, the PSA begins to rise to 15 and a bone scan now shows abnormal uptake in multiple ribs and the thoracic spine. Mr. Smith is started on an anti-androgen drug and his PSA drops to 10 at his 3-month followup visit. One year later his PSA has risen to 40, and he now says he has mild rib pain. Dr. Brown explains to Mr. Smith that he needs to consult with an oncologist from the cancer center, Dr. Mary Jones, and that Mr. Smith may need to see her. Mr. Smith somewhat reluctantly agrees to see Dr. Jones. Dr. Jones recommends exploring available clinical trials because Mr. Smith is young, is in good health with mild symptoms, and has a tumor that now appears to be progressing.

Finding a Clinical Trial

How can Dr. Brown or Dr. Jones find an appropriate clinical trial for Mr. Smith?

Dr. Jones decides to check NCI's PDQ system, because her center has no active trials for prostate cancer. The PDQ system will allow her to see current active clinical trials and their eligibility criteria. (For a further review of PDQ, please see section 6.)

Dr. Jones uses the NCI PDQ system to assess what, if any, clinical trials are available for Mr. Smith. Using the Internet, she accesses the site as follows:
- Enters the clinical trials section of *www.cancer.gov*
- Selects "Finding Clinical Trials"
- Selects PDQ Search Form
- Enters the relevant data; hits search (appropriate studies will be retrieved)
- Reviews the trials

If a physician does not have Internet access, how can he or she find a trial?

Clinical trial information is always available through NCI's Cancer Information Service (CIS) at 1-800-4-CANCER (1-800-422-6237).

After reviewing available trials, Dr. Jones selects a phase 2 trial entitled: *A Phase II Randomized Study of High–Dose Ketoconazole With or Without Alendronate Sodium in Patients With Androgen Independent Metastatic Adenocarcinoma of the Prostate* (2001) to discuss with Dr. Brown and Mr. Smith.

Mr. Smith is clinically eligible for the study. Participants are randomized to one of two arms: 1) a single oral dose of ketoconazole on day 1, and then 3 times daily oral dose beginning on day 8, versus 2) a single oral dose of alendronate sodium on day 1 and a single oral dose of ketoconazole on day 3 and then daily alendronate sodium and 3 times daily ketoconazole beginning on day 8. Participants who experience a clinically complete remission (CR) receive treatment for an additional 60 days beyond CR. Mr. Smith would have to be willing to have followup visits at NIH in Bethesda, MD, every 2 months and be seen in the NIH Cancer Center every 2 weeks for evaluation of toxicity and drug tolerance.

Sample Points to Discuss With the Patient Considering a Clinical Trial: Randomization, Patient Protection/Myths, and Insurance

Randomization

As a health care professional it is often challenging to discuss the concept of randomization with patients. Patients can feel threatened knowing that neither they, nor their doctor, can choose what treatment they will get if they enter a randomized trial. They may feel that the arm of the study that is standard care or closest to standard care, is the best option. People may also be concerned that if they enter a randomized clinical trial they will not receive treatment; they may receive just a "sugar pill." How can they be sure?

Dr. Jones began her discussion of randomization with Mr. Smith, his wife, and their two grown sons by explaining that this study has an objective group of professionals who monitor the study called a data and safety monitoring board (DMSB). The DMSB evaluates the data from the clinical trial to interpret if the therapy or technique being studied appears to be better (more beneficial) or worse (more harmful) than standard therapy. A trial can be halted early to allow all participants access to a clearly more beneficial intervention, or to protect participants from harm.

Dr. Jones explained that there are three phases for clinical trials and that randomization is generally seen in phase 3 studies where researchers are unsure whether a new intervention is better than the currently accepted standard therapy for a specific cancer type. She discussed how patients entering a phase 3 trial (and, as in this case, some phase 2 trials) are randomly assigned to groups (called randomization) and that neither the patients nor their doctors choose which therapy or technique they will receive. This is done because if physicians determined which therapy participants would receive, there could be an unconscious bias in their assignments. They could tend to assign patients with a more hopeful prognosis to the experimental therapy group and make the new therapy seem more effective than it really is. Similarly, if patients were allowed to choose which therapy they would receive, the results could also be influenced. Patients with a less hopeful prognosis could tend to pick the experimental treatment, for example, which may lead that treatment to look less effective than it really is.

Myths

Mr. Smith and his family have many questions regarding what they have heard and read about clinical trials. How would you answer these questions?

1. How do I know I am really safe if I enter this trial? You and I both know there are bad feelings in our community about research.

Fact: Tragedies have occurred in the past related to clinical trials. The African American community most notably remembers the infamous Tuskegee syphilis study, which followed, but did not treat, African American men with syphilis. There are now strong safeguards in place to protect research participants from the notorious human rights abuses of the past which include:

- Government oversight and regulations
- Institutional review board (IRB) review and approval of a clinical trial before it begins and annually while it is in progress
- An informed consent process which gives potential participants the information they need to decide about participation, including foreseeable risks and benefits
- Data and safety monitoring boards which ensure minimization of risks, integrity of trial data, and oversight to end a trial early if clear benefit or harm arises from the intervention being studied (usually used in phase 3 studies)

2. Aren't these clinical trials only for dying cancer patients?

Fact: Clinical trials are not just for patients with the most advanced disease. In fact, many newly diagnosed cancer patients participate in clinical trials. If only the sickest patients participated in treatment trials, researchers would not know how to treat patients with earlier stages of cancer. Phase 3 treatment includes all stages of cancer, from the most advanced to the most localized. These trials enroll hundreds or thousands of patients. Phase 1 and 2 cancer clinical trials, which enroll fewer than 100 patients, seek people with few treatment options or people who have exhausted all the current treatment options, which is Mr. Smith's case.

3. Aren't people who join clinical trials just "guinea pigs" for research?

Fact: People who decide to take part in a clinical trial are called participants, and strict guidelines are in place to ensure that these volunteers are treated as such:

- A participant has the right to withdraw from a trial at any time. The participant's decision does not jeopardize his or her future treatment and he or she may discuss further treatment options with the study physician or be referred back to a primary care provider for standard care.

- Although people fear that trial participants are treated like guinea pigs, reports from actual trial participants disagree. According to a Harris Poll conducted in 2000, the vast majority of trial participants said their overall experience was positive. Ninety-seven percent said they were treated with dignity and respect and that the quality of care they received was "excellent" or "good." More than 80 percent said they did not receive more tests than they felt were necessary and 86 percent said their treatment was covered by insurance.

4. Mr. Smith's wife is very concerned that cancer patients who join clinical treatment trials get a sugar pill (placebo) instead of really being treated. Will my husband really get treatment?

Fact: In phase 3 cancer treatment trials, participants with cancer get either a new treatment or the best standard treatment. In phase 2 trials, like the one Mr. Smith is considering, different schedules and combinations of two drugs are being evaluated for their effectiveness. It is unethical to deprive any person with a serious illness or condition of the best available treatment. There would be no placebo involved in Mr. Smith's treatment.

5. His oldest son is wondering if only people who have cancer can participate in a clinical trial. Aren't my brother and I at higher risk now?

Fact: Treatment and diagnostic trials are designed for people who already have cancer; however, genetics, prevention, and screening trials are designed for persons at risk of developing cancer. This is relevant for Mr. Smith's sons who now have an increased risk for prostate cancer. Dr. Jones suggests that the sons make an appointment to discuss a cancer prevention clinical trial.

Insurance

Dr. Brown is wondering whether participating in this cancer clinical trial will cost Mr. Smith more than standard treatment. Will insurance cover the costs?

The costs of new treatments for different cancers vary. Some treatments under study cost no more than standard therapies. Others, such as bone marrow transplants, are very expensive. There are hundreds of insurance companies and managed care organizations in the United States and each has a different policy about covering clinical trial costs. In general, most companies have contract language that prohibits coverage for "experimental therapies." However, decisions are often made on a case-by-case basis, and costs for patient care in clinical trials are often covered.

The best way to evaluate each situation is to ask questions such as the following:
- What will the total patient care costs be?
- What parts of the treatment, if any, does the study provide free of charge?
- What parts of treatment must be paid for by the participant or the participant's insurer?
- What is the situation for people who have no health insurance?
- Will total patient charges be higher for a clinical trial than for standard care?
- How often have insurers reimbursed all costs of the new therapy?
- Are there other resources or organizations that might help cover the fees or provide services, such as free transportation?

Another option is to discuss reimbursement issues with the insurance company ahead of time. The company is unlikely to promise coverage before the fact, but it may give information about general policies and trends. In considering costs of out-of-town treatment or follow-up care, patients should remember to include travel-related costs. The research team conducting the study will know how many times participants will need to visit, for how long, whether housing or stipends will be provided, and whether participants will be hospitalized during their stay.

Conclusion

After meeting with Dr. Jones and discussing their concerns, the Smith family met with Dr. Brown to discuss his view of the trial. Mr. Smith decided to enter the trial. After four months and his second evaluation, his PSA has decreased to 14 ng/ml, and he has no bone pain. He will continue for another cycle of therapy and be reevaluated in 2 months. After his initial apprehension eased and treatment began, Mr. Smith was able to verbalize satisfaction in both his decision to enter the trial and in the level of care and attention he received.

Glossary

adjuvant therapy: One or more anticancer drugs used in combination with surgery or radiation therapy as part of the treatment of cancer. Adjuvant therapy is given before or after the primary treatment to increase the chances of a cure. Adjuvant usually means "in addition to" initial treatment.

adverse effect: See *side effects*.

Adverse Event Expedited Reporting System: A Web-based program that enables researchers using NCI-sponsored investigational agents to expedite the reporting of serious and/or unexpected adverse events directly to NCI and FDA.

agent: In a cancer clinical trial, an agent is a substance that researchers believe might be capable of producing an effect that fights cancer.

assent: Children and adolescents are not deemed capable of giving true informed consent, so they are asked for their assent, or agreement, to participation in a clinical trial.

audit: In clinical trials, the onsite monitoring of trial procedures, documents, and data.

Belmont Report: A 1979 report by the National Commission for the Protection of Human Subjects of Biomedical and Behavioral Research that delineated the ethical principles upon which today's regulations regarding research participants in the United States are based: respect for persons, beneficence, and justice.

bias: Human choices, beliefs, or any other factors besides those being studied that affect a clinical trial's results. Clinical trials use many methods to avoid bias because biased results may not be correct.

biological therapy: Treatment to stimulate or restore the ability of the immune system to fight infection and disease. Also used to lessen side effects that may be caused by some cancer treatments. Also known as immunotherapy, biotherapy, or biological response modifier (BRM) therapy.

cancer: A term for diseases in which abnormal cells divide without control. Cancer cells can invade nearby tissues and can spread through the bloodstream and lymphatic system to other parts of the body.

cancer vaccine: A form of biological therapy, which may encourage a person's immune system to recognize cancer cells. These vaccines may help the body reject tumors and prevent cancer from recurring.

chemoprevention: The use of drugs, vitamins, or other agents to try to reduce the risk of, or delay the development or recurrence of, cancer.

chemotherapy: Treatment with anticancer drugs.

clinical trial: A research study that tests how well new medical treatments or other interventions work in people. Each study is designed to test new methods of screening, prevention, diagnosis, or treatment of a disease.

combination chemotherapy: Treatment using more than one anticancer drug.

combination therapy: The use of two or more modes of treatment—surgery, radiotherapy, chemotherapy, immunotherapy—in combination or alternately to achieve optimum results against cancer.

Common Toxicity Criteria: A Web-based, interactive application that uses standardized language to identify and grade adverse events in cancer clinical trials.

confidence intervals: These reflect a range of values surrounding the true score that would be obtained if everyone with a particular cancer were treated with the treatment under study. The wider the interval, the more variable the result and the less likely it is to be close to the true score. Confidence intervals are typically thought of as the approximate bounds or limits surrounding the true score. Researchers frequently use either a 95 or a 99 percent confidence interval.

control group: In a clinical trial, the group that receives the accepted standard treatment being studied. In cases where no standard treatment yet exists for a particular condition, the control group would receive no treatment. No patient is placed in a control group without treatment if there is any beneficial treatment known for that patient. This group is compared to the group that receives the investigational treatment. See also *investigational group*.

cooperative groups: Networks of institutions that jointly carry out large clinical trials following the same protocols.

data and safety monitoring board (DSMB): An independent committee whose membership includes, at minimum, a statistician and a clinical expert in the area being studied. Members may also include bioethicists or other clinicians knowledgeable about the trial's subject matter. The National Institutes of Health requires DSMB review of all phase 3 clinical trials. A DSMB might also review phase 1 or 2 trials that are blinded, take place at multiple locations, or employ particularly high-risk interventions or vulnerable populations.

diagnostic trial: A research study that evaluates methods of detecting disease.

disease-free survival: The amount of time a participant survives without cancer occurring or recurring, usually measured in months.

double-blinded: A clinical trial in which neither the medical staff nor the person knows which of several possible therapies the person is receiving.

eligibility criteria: Participant eligibility criteria for clinical trials can range from general (age, sex, type of cancer) to specific (prior treatment, tumor characteristics, blood cell counts, organ function). Eligibility criteria may also vary with trial phase. In phase 1 and 2 trials, the criteria often focus on making sure that people who might be harmed because of abnormal organ function or other factors are not put at risk. Phase 2 and 3 trials often add criteria regarding disease type and stage, and number of prior treatments.

endpoint: What researchers measure to evaluate the results of a new treatment being tested in a clinical trial. Research teams establish the endpoints of a trial before it begins. Examples of endpoints include *toxicity*, tumor response, survival time, and quality of life.

Food and Drug Administration (FDA): A consumer protection agency of the U.S. Department of Health and Human Services, FDA is required by law to review all test results for new drugs to ensure that they are safe and effective for specific uses.

gene: The functional and physical unit of heredity passed from parent to offspring. Genes are pieces of DNA, and most genes contain the information for making a specific protein.

gene therapy: Treatment that alters a gene. In studies of gene therapy for cancer, researchers are trying to improve the body's natural ability to fight the disease or to make the cancer cells more sensitive to other kinds of therapy.

genetic: Inherited; having to do with information that is passed from parents to offspring through genes in sperm and egg cells.

genetic epidemiologic research: Research that involves looking at tissue or blood samples from large populations of people in order to determine how one's genetic make-up can influence detection, diagnosis, prognosis, and ultimately, treatment.

genetics trials: Clinical trials that examine whether gene transfer therapy can be used to treat cancer, or whether genetic epidemiology research improves the understanding of cancer at the cellular level. Actual genetic intervention (such as gene transfer) trials are few in number, however trials are underway where actual cellular manipulation at the gene level occurs.

imaging: Tests that produce pictures of areas inside the body.

immunotherapy: See *biological therapy.*

informed consent: The process of providing all relevant information about the trial's purpose, risks, benefits, alternatives, and procedures to a potential participant, who then, consistent with his or her own interests and circumstances, makes an informed decision about whether to participate.

institutional review board (IRB): A board designed to oversee the research process in order to protect participant safety. Made up of researchers, ethicists, and laypeople from the community, the board must review the trial protocols and the informed consent forms participants sign.

intervention: The study agent or method that is being tested in a clinical trial or clinical study. The intervention is usually given to the investigational group while the control group receives standard treatment.

investigational group: In a clinical trial, the group that receives the new agent being tested. See also *control group.*

investigational new drug (IND): A drug that the Food and Drug Administration (FDA) allows to be used in clinical trials but that the FDA has not approved for commercial marketing.

metastasis: The spread of cancer from one part of the body to another. In cancer, metastasis is the migration of cancer cells from the original tumor site through the blood and lymph vessels to produce cancers in other tissues. Tumors formed from cells that have spread are called "secondary tumors" and contain cells that are like those in the original (primary) tumor. The plural is metastases.

metastatic cancer: Cancer that has spread from the place in which it started to other parts of the body.

monoclonal antibodies: Laboratory-produced substances that can locate and bind to cancer cells wherever they are in the body. Many monoclonal antibodies are used in cancer detection or therapy; each one recognizes a different protein on certain cancer cells. Monoclonal antibodies can be used alone, or they can be used to deliver drugs, toxins, or radioactive material directly to a tumor.

multimodality therapy: Therapy that combines more than one method of treatment.

National Cancer Institute (NCI): Part of the National Institutes of Health, of the United States Department of Health and Human Services, is the Federal Government's principal agency for cancer research. NCI conducts, coordinates, and funds cancer research, training, health information dissemination, and other programs with respect to the cause, diagnosis, prevention, and treatment of cancer. Access the NCI Web site at *www.cancer.gov.*

NCI-designated Cancer Centers: There are 3 kinds of NCI-designated cancer centers:
1. **Comprehensive cancer centers**, which conduct basic, clinical, and preventive research programs, as well as community outreach and education programs
2. **Clinical cancer centers**, which conduct primarily clinical research programs but may have programs in other research areas as well
3. **Cancer centers** (formerly called Basic Science Cancer Centers), which conduct basic or preventive research programs and do not have clinical programs

New Drug Application (NDA): The application filed with FDA by the trial sponsor once a trial has generated adequate data to support a certain indication for a drug.

Office for Human Research Protections (OHRP): Safeguards participants in federally funded research and provides unity and leadership for 17 Federal departments and agencies that carry out research involving human participants. OHRP enforces an important regulation called the Common Rule, which sets

CANCER CLINICAL TRIALS: THE IN-DEPTH PROGRAM

standards for the *informed consent* process; formation and function of *IRBs*; involvement of prisoners, children, and other vulnerable groups in research; and many other protective measures.

oncologist: A doctor who specializes in treating cancer. Some oncologists specialize in a particular type of cancer treatment. For example, a radiation oncologist specializes in treating cancer with radiation.

***p*-value:** A statistics term. A measure of probability that a difference between groups during an experiment happened by chance. For example, a *p*-value of .01 ($p = .01$) means there is a 1 in 100 chance the result occurred by chance. The smaller the *p*-value, the more likely it is that the difference between groups was caused by a difference between the tested treatments.

peer review: Scientific review by a panel of experts. The primary responsibility of these experts is to assess the scientific and technical merit of research proposals.

pharmacokinetics: The activity of drugs in the body over a period of time, including the processes by which drugs are absorbed, distributed in the body, localized in the tissues, and excreted.

phase 1 trial: Small groups of people with cancer are treated with a certain dose of a new agent that has already been extensively studied in the laboratory. During the trial, the dose is usually increased group by group in order to find the highest dose that does not cause harmful side effects. This process determines a safe and appropriate dose to use in a phase 2 trial.

phase 2 trial: Phase 2 trials continue to test the safety of the new agent and begin to evaluate how well it works against a specific type of cancer. In these trials, the new agent is given to groups of people with one type of cancer or related cancers, using the dosage found to be safe in phase 1 trials.

phase 3 trial: Phase 3 trials are designed to answer research questions across the disease continuum. Phase 3 trials usually have hundreds to thousands of participants, in order to find out if there are true differences in the effectiveness of the treatment being tested.

phase 4 trial: Phase 4 trials are used to evaluate the long-term safety and effectiveness of a treatment. Less common than phase 1, 2, and 3 trials, phase 4 trials take place after the new treatment has been approved for standard use.

Physician Data Query (PDQ®): PDQ is an online database developed and maintained by the National Cancer Institute. Designed to make the most current, credible, and accurate cancer information available to health professionals and the public, PDQ contains peer-reviewed summaries on cancer treatment, screening, prevention, genetics, and supportive care; a registry of cancer clinical trials from around the world; and directories of physicians, professionals who provide genetics services, and organizations that provide cancer care.

placebo: An inactive substance that looks the same as, and is administered in the same way as, a drug in a clinical trial. A placebo may be compared with a new drug when no one knows if any drug or treatment will be effective.

preclinical testing: A process in which scientists test promising new cancer treatments in the laboratory and in animal models. This is done to find out whether agents have an anticancer effect and are safely tolerated in animals. Once an agent proves promising in the lab, the sponsor applies for Food and Drug Administration approval to test it in clinical trials involving people.

prevention trials: Trials involving healthy people who are at high risk for developing cancer. These trials try to answer specific questions about and evaluate the effectiveness of ways to reduce the risk of cancer.

principal investigator: The person responsible for overseeing all aspects of a clinical trial, specifically, for developing the concept and writing the protocol; submitting the protocol for institutional review board approval; recruiting participants; obtaining informed consent; and collecting, analyzing, interpreting, and presenting data.

protocol: A written, detailed action plan for a clinical trial. The protocol provides the background, specifies the objectives, and describes the design and organization of the trial. Every center participating in the trial uses the same protocol, ensuring consistency of procedures and enhancing communication among everyone working on the trial. This uniformity ensures that participant information from all centers can be combined and compared.

quality of life: The overall enjoyment of life. Many clinical trials measure aspects of an individual's sense of well-being and ability to perform various tasks to assess the effects of cancer and its treatment on the overall quality of life.

radiation therapy: The use of high-energy radiation from x-rays, gamma rays, neutrons, and other sources to kill cancer cells and shrink tumors. Radiation may come from a machine outside the body (external-beam radiation therapy), or it may come from radioactive material placed in the body in the area near cancer cells (internal radiation therapy, implant radiation, or brachytherapy). Systemic radiation therapy uses a radioactive substance, such as a radiolabeled monoclonal antibody, that circulates throughout the body. Also called radiotherapy.

randomization: A method used to prevent bias in research. A computer or a table of random numbers generates treatment assignments, and participants have an equal chance to be assigned to one of two or more groups (e.g., the *control group* or the *investigational group*).

randomized clinical trial: A study in which the participants are assigned by chance to separate groups that compare different treatments; neither the researchers nor the participants can choose which group. Using chance to assign people to groups means that the groups will be similar and that the treatments they receive can be compared objectively. At the time of the trial, it is not known which treatment is best. It is the patient's choice to be in a randomized trial.

recurrence: The return of cancer, at the same site as the original (primary) tumor or in another location, after the tumor had disappeared.

regimen: A treatment plan that specifies the dosage, the schedule, and the duration of treatment.

regression: A decrease in the size of a tumor, or in the extent of cancer in the body.

relative risk: In cancer treatment trials, the likelihood that cancer will recur within a specific timeframe in one intervention group versus another.

remission: A decrease in or disappearance of signs and symptoms of cancer. In partial remission, some, but not all, signs and symptoms of cancer have disappeared. In complete remission, all signs and symptoms of cancer have disappeared, although there still may be cancer in the body.

risk/benefit ratio: The relation between the risks and benefits of a given treatment or procedure. An *institutional review board*, usually located where the clinical trial is to take place, determines whether the risks in the trial are reasonable with respect to the potential benefits. It is up to individual potential participants to decide whether it is reasonable for them in particular to participate.

sample size: In clinical trials, the number of people participating in a trial.

screening trials: Clinical trials that assess the effectiveness of new means of detecting cancer early in healthy people, especially the earliest stages of cancer. For many types of cancer, early detection results in improved outcomes. In addition, these trials examine whether early treatment, as a result of early detection, actually improves overall survival or disease-free survival.

side effects: Problems that occur when treatment affects healthy cells. Common side effects of cancer treatment are fatigue, nausea, vomiting, decreased blood cell counts, hair loss, and mouth sores.

single-blinded: Describes clinical trials set up in such a way that participants do not know which therapy or intervention they are receiving.

stage: The extent of a cancer, especially whether the disease has spread from the original site to other parts of the body. Numbers with or without letters are used to define cancer stages (e.g., stage IIb).

standard treatment: A currently accepted and widely used treatment for a certain type of cancer, based on the results of past research.

statistical power: The chance of getting a *statistically significant* result when there is one. Ideally, in clinical trials statistical power should be .80 or .90—in other words, there is an 80 to 90 percent chance that the true difference in effectiveness between the treatments is the smallest size considered medically important to detect.

statistically significant: Describes a mathematical measure of difference between groups. The difference is said to be statistically significant if it is greater than what might be expected to happen by chance alone.

stratification: A separation process used in randomized trials when factors that can influence the intervention's success are known. For example, participants whose cancer has spread from the original tumor site can be separated, or stratified, from those whose cancer has not spread. Assignment of interventions within the two groups is then randomized. Stratification enables researchers to look in separate subgroups to see whether differences exist.

toxicity: Harmful side effects from an *agent* being tested.

treatment group: See *investigational group* and *control group*.

treatment trials: Treatment trials are designed to test the safety and effectiveness of new drugs, biological agents, techniques, or other interventions in people who have been diagnosed with cancer. These trials evaluate the novel treatment against standard treatment, if there is one.

tumor: An abnormal mass of tissue that results from excessive cell division. Tumors perform no useful body function. They may be benign (not cancerous) or malignant (cancerous).

vaccine: A substance or group of substances meant to cause the immune system to respond to a cancer or to microorganisms, such as bacteria or viruses.

Bibliography

American Cancer Society. (2002). *Cancer facts and figures.* Atlanta, GA.

Barrett, R. (2002). A nurse's primer on recruiting participants for clinical trials. *Oncology Nursing Forum*, 29(7), 1091-1098.

Bennett, C.L., Stinson, T. J., Vogel, V., Robertson, L., Leedy, D., O'Brien, P., Hobbs, J., Sutton, T., Ruckdeschel, J. C., Chirikos, T. N., Weiner, R. S., Ramsey, M. M., & Wicha, M. S. (2000). Evaluating the financial impact of clinical trials in oncology: Results from a pilot study from the Association of American Cancer Institutes/Northwestern University Clinical Trials Costs and Charges Project. *Journal of Clinical Oncology*, 18, 2805-2810.

Fireman, B., Fehrenbacher, L., Gruskin, E. P., & Ray, G. T. (2000). Cost of care for patients in cancer clinical trials. *Journal of the National Cancer Institute*, 92, 136-142.

Food and Drug Administration. (2001). *www.fda.gov* [Web site].

Harris Interactive. (2001). *Health Care News*, 1(3). [Poll]. Available from *http://harrisinteractive.com/about/healthnews/HI_HealthCareNews2001 Vol_iss3.pdf*

Klimaszewski, A., Aikin, J., Bacon, M., DiStasio, S., Ehrenberger, H., & Ford, B. (Eds.). (2000). *Manual for clinical trials nursing.* Pittsburgh, PA: Oncology Nursing Press.

National Cancer Institute. (2001). *http://cancernet.nci.nih.gov* [Web site].

National Cancer Institute. (2001). *http://cancernet.nci.nih.gov/cancerlit.html* [Web site].

National Cancer Institute. (2001). *http://cancertrials.nci.nih.gov* [Web site].

National Cancer Institute. (2001). *http://ctep.info.nih.gov* [Web site].

Shalala, D. (2000). Protecting research subjects—What must be done. *New England Journal of Medicine, 343,* 808-810.

Wagner, J. L., Alberts, S. R., Sloan, J. A., Cha, S., Killian, J., O'Connell, M. J., Van Grevenhof, P., Lindman, J., & Chute, C. G. (1999). Incremental costs of enrolling cancer patients in clinical trials: A population-based study. *Journal of the National Cancer Institute, 91,* 847-853.